Clean Eating Cookbook fo

A 1200-Day Journey of Nurturing Mind and Body with Simple,
Delicious Recipes for You and Your Family + Bonus:
Comprehensive 30-Day Meal Plan

Kaylee Anderson

Table of Contents

1. Introduction

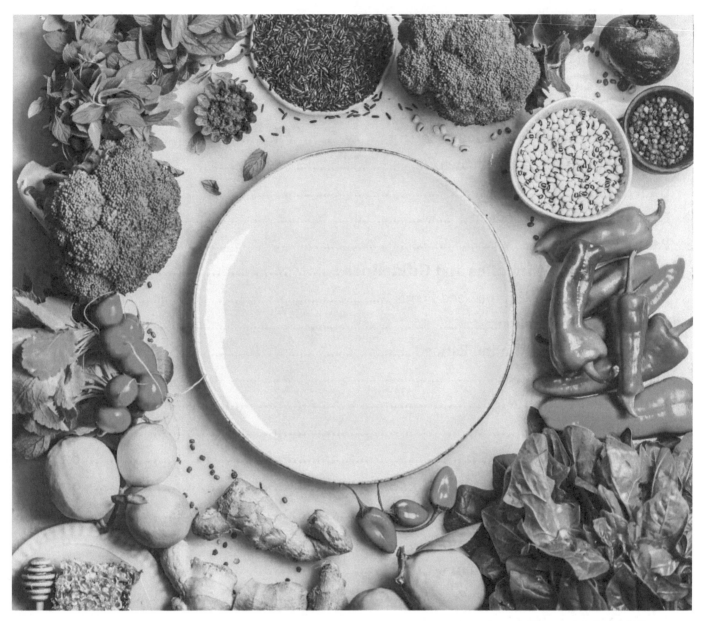

Philosophy of Clean Eating

The philosophy of clean eating, a concept deeply rooted in the principles of nourishment and purity, advocates for a lifestyle approach that emphasizes the holistic consumption of minimally processed foods, aiming to maximize the body's intake of essential nutrients while simultaneously minimizing exposure to the potentially harmful substances prevalent in processed foods. This approach is not just about the food itself but also its journey from source to plate, necessitating a conscious awareness of each stage of a food's production and processing. It champions the consumption of items that remain as close to their natural, unaltered state as possible, operating under the premise that these foods are more in sync with the body's natural biological processes, thereby promoting better overall health and well-being.

Moreover, clean eating is an ethos that extends its concern to environmental sustainability, advocating for the prioritization of locally sourced produce and products created through environmentally friendly methods, effectively reducing the carbon footprint linked to long-distance food transportation and detrimental agricultural practices. This philosophy doesn't exist in isolation but intersects significantly with ethical considerations, promoting choices that reflect a responsibility not just to personal health but also to the broader social and environmental contexts. It transcends the narrow focus on weight loss or aesthetics, instead endorsing a comprehensive view that acknowledges food as a crucial determinant of one's quality of life, with profound implications for physical health, mental clarity, and even lifespan.

Additionally, clean eating encourages a mindfulness that transforms one's dietary habits, necessitating deliberate and informed choices that extend beyond mere ingestion to a deeper understanding of food's impact on physical health, mental states, and emotional well-being. This mindfulness, cultivated through a focus on whole, unprocessed foods, fosters a heightened bodily awareness and a nuanced understanding of the immediate and long-term effects of food consumption.

In practical terms, adherence to this philosophy manifests in daily habits and dietary choices characterized by scrutinizing food labels to avoid harmful or artificial ingredients, opting for whole grains over their refined counterparts, prioritizing lean proteins, and ensuring a diet rich in a diverse array of fruits and vegetables. It also necessitates the limitation of added sugars and salt, with a preference for water as the primary beverage.

In essence, the philosophy of clean eating represents a commitment that extends beyond the individual, touching on communal and environmental health. It's an all-encompassing approach demanding not just awareness and intentionality in dietary choices, but also a profound desire to cultivate a lifestyle marked by health, balance, and holistic well-being.

Benefits of Clean Eating

The benefits of clean eating significantly influence health and well-being, starting with enhanced general health; consuming foods in their natural state ensures the body receives essential nutrients, fostering good health, robust immune function, and efficient organ operation. These whole foods are replete with crucial vitamins, minerals, and antioxidants, mitigating the risk of chronic ailments such as heart disease, diabetes, and cancer. Additionally, the avoidance of processed foods, notorious for high refined sugar and carbohydrate content, eliminates the energy spikes and subsequent crashes, commonly culminating in fatigue. Instead, clean eating stabilizes energy levels, with numerous reports of heightened mental clarity and concentration. Weight management is another advantage, as the high unhealthy fats and sugars in processed foods contribute to weight gain, whereas a whole food diet provides a balanced nutrient intake, facilitating weight control. Furthermore, the dietary fiber in whole foods like grains, fruits, and vegetables bolsters digestive health, essential for regular bowel movements and a healthy gut microbiome, both integral to overall health.

Clean eating also combats chronic inflammation, a contributor to numerous severe illnesses, by emphasizing a diet rich in fruits, vegetables, and omega-3 fatty acids, known for their inflammation-reducing antioxidants. This approach impacts emotional health, with many noting feelings of calm, happiness, and reduced anxiety with improved diet. There's also a positive correlation between clean eating and sleep quality, especially when the diet includes foods rich in nutrients like calcium, magnesium, and vitamin D. In the broader scope, clean eating potentially extends life expectancy by lowering chronic disease risk, aiding weight maintenance, and enhancing overall health. Environmentally, it advocates for locally sourced, organic foods, reducing the carbon footprint linked to food production and transport, while economically, despite higher upfront costs, it can lead to long-term savings by reducing healthcare expenses related to chronic diseases and other health complications. In essence, clean eating's benefits are multifaceted, improving physical and mental health, and contributing to environmental and economic well-being, underscoring its role in fostering a healthier, higher quality of life.

How to Transition to Clean Eating

Transitioning to clean eating is a gradual, transformative journey that necessitates comprehension, strategic planning, and a steadfast commitment to healthier culinary selections. The initial, critical step involves a thorough understanding of clean eating, a concept emphasizing the consumption of whole, minimally processed foods, and a comprehensive grasp of the nutritional merits of diverse foodstuffs. This entails an educational deep dive into the realm of food labels, ingredient lists, and nutritional data, equipping oneself with the knowledge to sidestep ostensibly healthy but actually deleterious foods, often concealed behind veils of sugars, unhealthy fats, or preservatives.

Embarking on this journey doesn't demand an abrupt, comprehensive dietary revamp; rather, it advocates for incremental changes. This could mean incorporating an increased quantity of fruits and vegetables into your diet, preferring whole grains to their refined counterparts, or selecting lean proteins, concurrently curtailing the consumption of processed items, sugary drinks, and fatty snacks.

Strategic meal planning emerges as a cornerstone in this transition, necessitating a weekly meal blueprint and corresponding grocery list, a tactic that fortifies one's resolve to adhere to dietary aspirations while diminishing the allure of impromptu dining out or ordering in. It's imperative that this plan encompasses a diverse array of foods, guaranteeing a balanced nutritional intake.

The ethos of clean eating transcends the mere content of your meals, extending to a mindful appreciation of each culinary experience. This involves attentiveness to natural hunger signals, a leisurely eating pace, and a conscious savoring of every bite, enhancing not only the gastronomic experience but also precluding overindulgence. Hydration, often sidelined, plays a crucial role; adequate water intake facilitates digestion, sustains energy, and can even mitigate the likelihood of mistaking thirst for hunger.

The journey is seldom solitary; seeking support from communal sources, be they relatives, acquaintances, or digital cohorts, can significantly smoothen the transition. Patience and flexibility are indispensable, acknowledging that this transformative journey will present challenges and necessitate time. Learning from these hurdles and persisting, while allowing for occasional indulgences, aligns with the holistic ethos of clean eating.

Clean eating, far from a finite goal, is an ongoing journey of informed, health-conscious decisions, acknowledging the profound influence of our dietary choices on our holistic health, well-being, and life quality.

2. Getting Started with Clean Eating

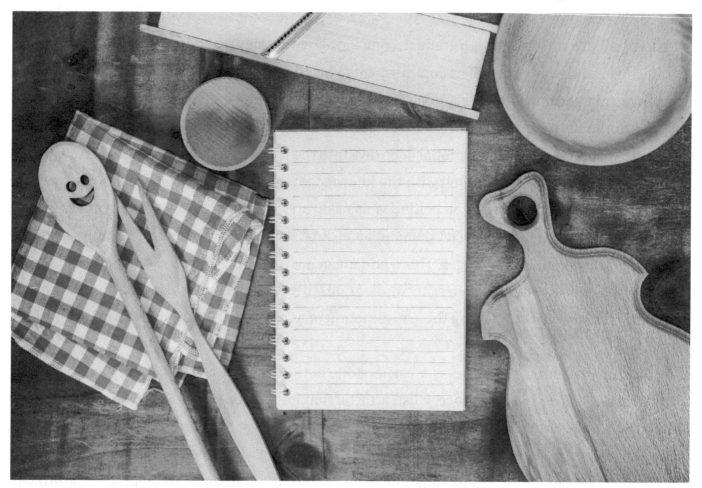

Setting up a Clean Eating Kitchen

Setting up a clean eating kitchen requires a holistic approach, starting with purging unhealthy items to eliminate temptations, thereby making room for essential clean eating staples like fresh fruits, vegetables, whole grains, lean proteins, and healthy fats. Organization is key; arranging the kitchen so that healthy options are more accessible and visible can encourage better eating habits, while investing in quality cookware and safe, BPA-free food storage containers can enhance the meal preparation experience and ensure food safety. Visible meal plans can serve as daily reminders and motivation, and having a list of healthy recipes can provide quick solutions on busy days. It's also important to involve and educate household members about the benefits of clean eating, fostering a supportive environment. Regular evaluation of kitchen stocks and eating habits is necessary for sustained adherence to this lifestyle, accommodating changing needs and preferences. Integrating sustainability practices, such as buying local produce and using eco-friendly products, aligns the clean eating lifestyle with environmental consciousness. Additionally, creating a mindful atmosphere in the kitchen, perhaps through calming music or natural decor, can make the space more inviting and reinforce a positive relationship with food. This comprehensive setup ensures not just a kitchen conducive to clean eating but also promotes an overall lifestyle that supports health and well-being.

KITCHEN CONVERSIONS

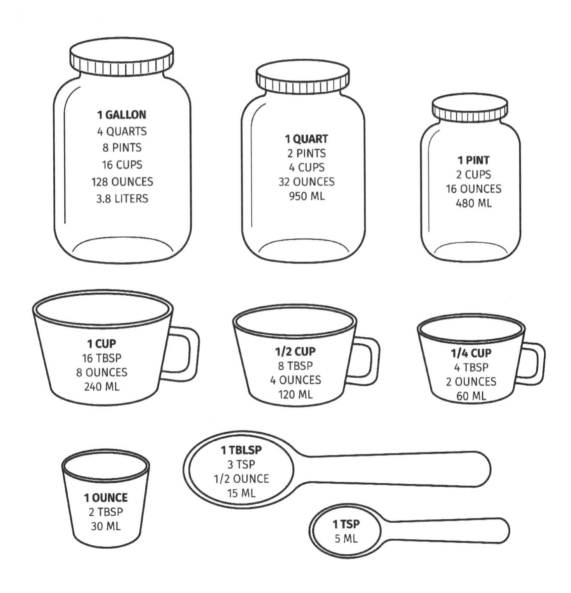

1 GALLON
4 QUARTS
8 PINTS
16 CUPS
128 OUNCES
3.8 LITERS

1 QUART
2 PINTS
4 CUPS
32 OUNCES
950 ML

1 PINT
2 CUPS
16 OUNCES
480 ML

1 CUP
16 TBSP
8 OUNCES
240 ML

1/2 CUP
8 TBSP
4 OUNCES
120 ML

1/4 CUP
4 TBSP
2 OUNCES
60 ML

1 OUNCE
2 TBSP
30 ML

1 TBLSP
3 TSP
1/2 OUNCE
15 ML

1 TSP
5 ML

Understanding Food Labels

Mastering the art of interpreting food labels is indispensable in the journey of clean eating, serving as the compass that guides individuals through the labyrinth of choices present in the food market. At the heart of this deciphering process is the ingredients list, presented in a descending order of predominance. Advocates of clean eating gravitate towards products with succinct lists comprising familiar, unadulterated ingredients, while maintaining a vigilant eye out for red flags such as artificial additives or preservatives.

Equally crucial is the comprehension of serving sizes and the total number of servings per container, which serve as the yardstick for calibrating one's consumption of calories and other nutrients. The nutritional section of the label serves as a beacon, illuminating the quantities of integral components like fats, cholesterol, sodium, carbohydrates, fibers, sugars, and proteins. The clean eating doctrine champions a diet lower in saturated fats, cholesterol, and sodium, while celebrating the virtues of dietary fiber.

The Percent Daily Values (%DV) act as a nutritional barometer, reflecting the percentage of daily recommended nutrient quotas contained in a single serving, predicated on a standard 2,000-calorie diet, thereby facilitating a food's nutritional assessment within the broader narrative of one's entire dietary intake. Moreover, nutrient content claims, such as "low sodium" or "rich in fiber," are not mere marketing ploys but are tethered to FDA regulations, offering a snapshot of a food's nutritional profile.

For those navigating the dietary restrictions imposed by food allergies or sensitivities, allergen information is a lighthouse, typically nestled at the conclusion of the ingredient list, signaling the presence of ubiquitous allergens. In the clean eating universe, labels such as "organic" or "non-GMO" are not just accolades but affirmations of compliance with stringent USDA guidelines, including freedom from synthetic pesticides, artificial fertilizers, and bioengineered genes. Expiration dates, while not definitive arbiters of safety, are nonetheless vital signposts for quality and freshness. Additionally, the country of origin of a product, though often overlooked, resonates with significance for proponents of local sourcing as a means to mitigate environmental strain and bolster local commerce.

In essence, the ability to decode food labels is less a skill and more a survival tool, a critical conduit to making enlightened food choices that resonate with one's health objectives and the principles of clean eating. It demands meticulous attention and an informed perspective on one's nutritional requisites, acting as the bedrock upon which the edifice of clean eating is erected.

Essential Kitchen Equipment

Embarking on the clean eating journey is significantly streamlined with the arsenal of appropriate kitchen equipment, acting as invaluable allies in concocting fresh, nutrient-packed meals. The cornerstone of this culinary battalion is a suite of high-caliber knives, encompassing a versatile chef's knife for routine chopping, a serrated knife adept at slicing through bread and tomatoes with minimal waste, and a nimble paring knife for intricate tasks like peeling or fine slicing. Complementing this cutting-edge trio are multiple cutting boards, a strategic move to thwart cross-contamination between fresh produce and various raw meats, with materials such as bamboo marrying ease of cleaning with kindness to your knives' sharpness.

In the realm of electric appliances, the blender stands as a multifaceted champion, facilitating the seamless integration of fruits, vegetables, and nuts into one's diet through its prowess in whipping up smoothies, soups, and sauces. Its culinary cousin, the food processor, is a godsend for time-efficient preparation, making light work of laborious tasks like chopping, dicing, and even dough preparation. Steamer baskets, with their nutrient-conserving mode of cooking, represent a simplistic yet potent tool, compatible with existing pots and invaluable for their ability to preserve the nutritional integrity of food.

The humble slow cooker, celebrated for its proficiency in batch cooking, shines in its ability to meld flavors over extended periods, negating the need for excess fats while safeguarding moisture and nutrient content.

Precision in culinary arts is afforded by the unassuming yet essential measuring cups and spoons, critical for adhering to portion sizes and ensuring recipe accuracy. The sanctity of clean eating extends to the realm of cookware; non-toxic variants like cast iron, stainless steel, and ceramic are revered for their inert nature, preventing any chemical migration to your meals. Additional gadgets like a salad spinner, vegetable spiralizer, and mortar and pestle facilitate the regular incorporation of fresh salads, provide healthy substitutes to pasta, and allow for the creation of preservative-free seasonings, respectively.

A digital kitchen scale, often overlooked, is instrumental for portion-conscious individuals, delivering precise ingredient quantification. Lastly, the journey of clean eating transcends solid food, advocating for the purity of water consumption. This compendium of kitchen apparatus, far from mere gadgets, paves the way for a seamless, enjoyable transition to clean eating, equipping you with the means to craft an array of palatable, nourishing meals that resonate with the ethos of clean eating.

Pantry Essentials

A well-stocked pantry is the cornerstone of clean eating, brimming with natural, unprocessed ingredients that are the bedrock of a nourishing diet. Whole grains like quinoa, brown rice, and various whole wheat or legume-based pastas, not forgetting barley and oats, are indispensable, offering a rich tapestry of fiber, vitamins, and minerals, and serving as a wholesome foundation for an array of dishes. Legumes, encompassing beans, lentils, and chickpeas, are celebrated for their hearty protein content and fiber richness, making them a versatile ally in everything from robust salads to comforting soups and stews. Nuts and seeds, with their cadre of almonds, walnuts, chia seeds, flaxseeds, and pumpkin seeds, are a treasure trove of healthy fats, protein, and fiber, doubling as convenient snacks, crunchy salad garnishes, or nutritious additions to breakfast bowls. The triumvirate of healthy oils - extra virgin olive oil, coconut oil, and avocado oil - are the heart-healthy quintessence of fats, indispensable in cooking and concocting dressings. Dried or canned fruits, used judiciously, serve as natural sweetening agents in various dishes or as standalone snacks, especially those devoid of added sugars or sulfites.

The culinary world owes much of its vibrancy to spices and herbs; whether fresh or dried, they infuse dishes with a burst of flavor sans extra calories or sodium, with stalwarts like garlic, turmeric, cumin, rosemary, and thyme being pantry mainstays. Vinegars, particularly balsamic varieties, are flavor powerhouses, especially in homemade salad dressings. When the need for sweetness arises, natural sweeteners such as honey, maple syrup, or stevia step in, offering a touch of sweetness without resorting to refined sugars.

Nut butters, spanning almond, peanut, and cashew varieties, emerge as snack-time champions and are delightful inclusions in smoothies or oatmeal, provided they are free of added sugars or hydrogenated oils. The realm of plant-based milks presents lactose-free alternatives like almond, coconut, or oat milk, while quick protein sources manifest in canned or dried legumes, natural nut butters, unsalted nuts, and seeds.

Whole grain flours, including coconut, almond, or whole wheat varieties, offer healthier avenues for baking enthusiasts. Low-sodium broths, whether vegetable, chicken, or beef, form the soul of soups and stews, with a preference for organic varieties.

Sea salt emerges as a more wholesome seasoning alternative, used sparingly, while the availability of pre-washed greens is a subtle encouragement for frequent salad indulgence. Equipped with these clean eating stalwarts, you're poised to craft nutrient-dense, healthful meals and snacks, fortifying your wellness journey.

3. Clean Eating Principles and Guidelines

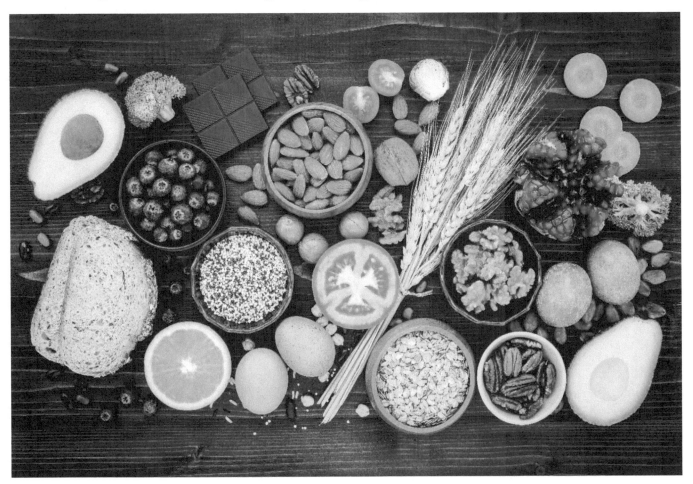

Focusing on Whole, Unprocessed Foods

Focusing on whole, unprocessed foods, a cornerstone of clean eating, involves consuming foods in their natural state or minimally processed, offering numerous health benefits. These foods, including fresh fruits, vegetables, whole grains, lean proteins, and nuts, are nutrient-dense, providing essential vitamins, minerals, and antioxidants crucial for optimal health and protection against diseases like diabetes, heart disease, and cancer. Unlike processed foods, whole foods are free from harmful additives, preservatives, and artificial ingredients that can negatively impact health, potentially leading to weight gain, metabolic issues, and an increased risk of various conditions. They're typically lower in calories, helping in weight management, and provide dietary fiber, essential for digestive health, blood sugar regulation, heart health, and reduced risk of chronic diseases. Additionally, they promote satiety, helping control appetite and food intake. However, this dietary shift isn't without challenges; it demands planning, meal preparation, understanding of nutrition, and cooking skills.

Importance of Hydration

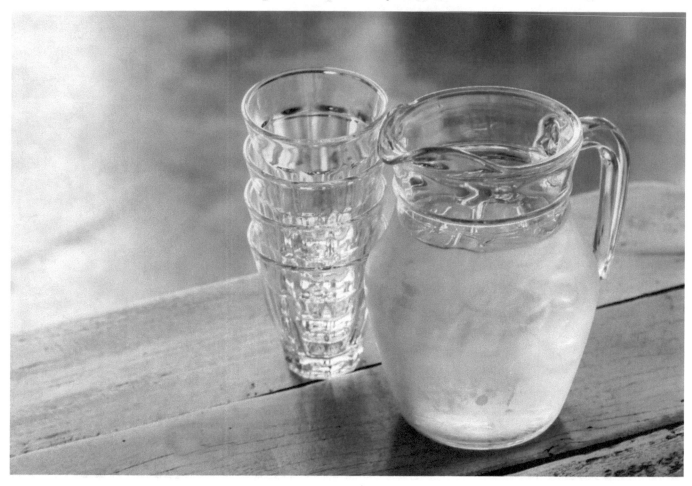

The quintessence of hydration within the clean eating ethos is irrefutable, given water's cardinal role in a plethora of physiological functions and overarching health. As the human body's most profuse molecule, water constitutes approximately 60% of an adult's body weight, serving as an irreplaceable component for cellular equilibrium and the seamless operation of every bodily system, encompassing the circulatory, respiratory, and neurological spheres.

Primarily, water is the linchpin in sustaining the equilibrium of bodily fluids, which are instrumental in a myriad of processes including digestion, absorption, circulation, saliva production, nutrient transportation, and thermoregulation. When fluid levels dwindle, the brain instigates the body's thirst mechanism — a signal of paramount importance, not to be dismissed, as unwavering hydration is imperative for the efficacious functioning of these physiological processes.

The realm of physical performance is not impervious to hydration's influence. Physical exertion precipitates water loss via perspiration, and a deficit in fluid replenishment can spiral into dehydration, markedly impairing physical capabilities. This state manifests in escalated fatigue, plummeting motivation, an amplified sense of effort, and a predisposition to overheating. Diligent hydration can forestall these repercussions, optimizing performance during physical endeavors and curtailing oxidative stress during strenuous activities.

In the context of renal function, water's significance is pronounced. Kidneys, the arbiters of bodily fluid regulation, rely on adequate water consumption to expel sodium, urea, and toxins, thwarting their accumulation and subsequent renal impairment. Persistent dehydration can culminate in renal lithiasis and other kidney afflictions.

Skin health and aesthetics, too, are tethered to hydration. A paucity of water can render skin parched and accentuate wrinkles, whereas adequate hydration can rejuvenate the skin's appearance. Nonetheless, it's prudent to acknowledge that superfluous hydration won't efface established wrinkles or fine lines.

Hydration also emerges as a cornerstone in weight regulation and reduction strategies. The body, in its complexity, can misconstrue thirst for hunger, inciting excessive caloric consumption when the actual demand is for water. Imbibing water pre-meals can engender satiety and temper appetite, averting excessive food intake. Furthermore, water's caloric absence renders it an optimal hydration source, devoid of the sugars and additives rampant in numerous commercial beverages.

Within clean eating parameters, water reigns supreme as the beverage par excellence, untainted by the additives, sugars, and preservatives that besiege sodas, sports concoctions, and other processed libations. This preference mirrors the clean eating tenet of ingesting edibles and potables in their purest form.

However, water requirements fluctuate, influenced by variables such as climatic conditions, the intensity of physical activity, and personal health nuances. The oft-cited guideline — consuming eight 8-ounce glasses of water daily — stands as a sensible benchmark, albeit the actual quantum may oscillate, necessitating more or less. It's pertinent to note that total water intake encompasses not just beverages but also the moisture innate in foods, particularly fruits and vegetables.

In summation, optimal hydration is a health imperative, with far-reaching effects spanning physical performance, metabolic processes, renal functionality, and weight stewardship. Within the clean eating doctrine, it underscores the devotion to natural, salubrious substances while eschewing processed, potentially deleterious alternatives.

Portion Control and Mindful Eating

Portion control and mindful eating stand as pillars in the clean eating doctrine, underscoring the importance of not just the calibre of food consumed, but also the quantity and the awareness accompanying its consumption. These practices are indispensable in sustaining a healthy weight, averting overconsumption, and guaranteeing the body assimilates necessary nutrients without the surplus calories that potentially precipitate weight augmentation and health complications. Portion control revolves around comprehending and allocating appropriate food quantities, a strategy that tempers calorie intake and is pivotal for individuals aspiring to healthily lose, sustain, or increase weight. Erroneous portion size estimations can culminate in overeating, even when the food is inherently healthy. Effective portion control strategies encompass utilizing smaller plates, quantifying servings, deciphering food labels, and heeding innate hunger signals. Conversely, mindful eating is an exercise in heightening one's consciousness regarding eating habits, instilling a pause between triggers and actions, and necessitating undivided attention to the multifaceted experience of eating and drinking. This involves cognizance of sensory stimuli — taste, aroma, consistency — and emotional reactions, eating deliberately in the absence of distractions, interpreting physical hunger cues, differentiating genuine hunger from unrelated triggers, engaging senses by observing colors, scents, sounds, textures, and tastes, and managing feelings of guilt or anxiety associated with food.

These practices are not mutually exclusive but rather intricately linked. Mindful eating fosters a natural propensity for portion control, as it hones one's sensitivity to the body's hunger and fullness signals, thereby circumventing overconsumption, subsequent discomfort, and potential chronic health ramifications ensuing from excessive caloric intake. Nevertheless, the implications of these practices transcend weight regulation, contributing to enhanced digestion — as leisurely eating and thorough mastication ameliorate symptoms linked to digestive ailments — and augmenting the culinary experience by encouraging the savoring of meals.

The integration of portion control and mindful eating into one's daily regime doesn't equate to dieting in the traditional sense. Rather, it signifies the embracement of salubrious eating habits conducive to enduring modifications and amplified well-being. These methodologies advocate a harmonious rapport with food, preventing its demonization or utilization as an emotional prop.

Clean Eating on a Budget

Clean eating on a budget, contrary to popular belief, is an attainable and sustainable endeavor, necessitating meticulous planning, astute shopping, and adept food preparation. The notion that clean eating is exorbitantly costly is a misapprehension; indeed, through judicious strategies, one can indulge in a diet rich in clean, whole foods without draining one's finances.

Foremost, the cornerstone of economical clean eating is proficient meal planning. This involves an initial inventory check of existing supplies in your pantry, refrigerator, and freezer, followed by strategizing meals that incorporate these items, and finally, creating a precise shopping list to adhere to, thereby circumventing impulsive buys that tend to inflate expenses.

Opting for seasonal and locally-sourced produce significantly trims grocery bills, as these items are typically priced lower, fresher, and brimming with nutrients compared to out-of-season counterparts.

Purchasing in bulk proves cost-efficient for non-perishable or staple items, with whole grains, legumes, nuts, and seeds often available in large quantities at discounted rates.

Prioritizing whole foods and home-cooked meals over processed variants is financially and health-wise prudent; processed items, albeit cheap at first glance, lack in nutritional value and satiety, leading to increased consumption over time. In contrast, fiber-rich whole foods and home-prepared meals ensure nutritional adequacy, satisfaction, and more controlled spending.

Protein, often the priciest on the list, demands smart choices. Plant-based proteins such as beans, lentils, tofu, and tempeh are not only nutritious but also lighter on the wallet. For meat consumers, opting for less pricey cuts, buying in bulk, and efficient freezing can lead to substantial savings.

Minimizing food wastage is another crucial aspect.

Lastly, adept food preparation and storage, especially post bulk purchases, is key. This entails prepping meals in advance, portioning, and freezing for future consumption, which curbs spending and the lure of unhealthier, pricier alternatives.

In essence, clean eating need not be financially burdensome. It hinges on informed decision-making, preemptive planning, and inventive culinary approaches. By heeding these tips, one can maintain a nourishing dietary regimen that is both economically and physically health-sustaining.

4. Breakfast Delights

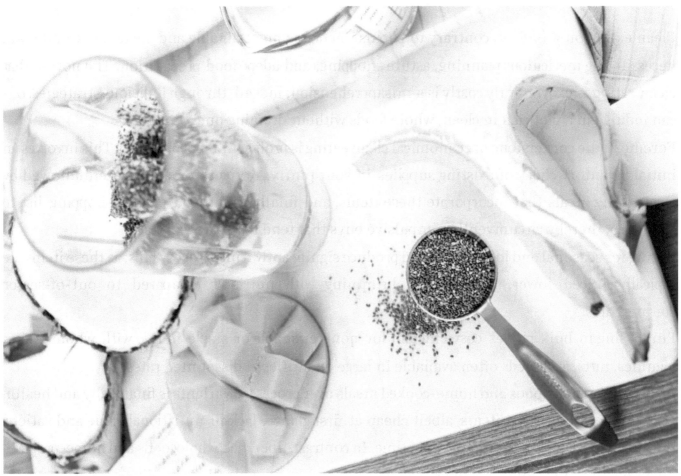

Mango Coconut Smoothie – Page 25

Let's dive into the invigorating world of clean eating, starting with the most important meal of the day: breakfast. This initial feast is fundamental, not just to fuel the body after a night's rest, but also to set the tone for the nourishment you'll provide your body throughout the day. In the realm of clean eating, breakfast isn't just a meal; it's an opportunity to infuse your body with unprocessed, whole foods that are as close to their natural state as possible.

Clean eating breakfasts embrace the simplicity and the flavors of each ingredient, creating a symphony of tastes and textures in every bite. It's about unearthing the joy in each meal, knowing that you're nourishing your body, mind, and soul with every forkful. So, begin your day with the purity and goodness of clean eating, and let this practice of mindfulness extend to every aspect of your life.

Sunrise Smoothie Bowl

Preparation Time:	Cooking Time:	Servings:
10 minutes	0 minutes	2

Ingredients:

1 cup mixed berries (strawberries, blueberries, raspberries)

1 banana, sliced

1 cup spinach leaves

1 tbsp chia seeds

1 cup almond milk, unsweetened

½ cup granola, no added sugar

2 tbsp coconut flakes, unsweetened

Instructions:

Blend mixed berries, banana, spinach leaves, chia seeds, and almond milk until smooth.

Pour the smoothie into bowls and top with granola and coconut flakes.

Nutritional Information (per serving):

Calories: 220	Carbs: 36g
Protein: 6g	Fat: 8g

Notes

_____
_____
_____
_____
_____
_____

Energizing Oat Pancakes

Preparation Time:

15 minutes

Cooking Time:

10 minutes

Servings:

2

Ingredients:

1 cup rolled oats

1 banana, mashed

2 eggs

½ tsp baking powder

1 tbsp honey

½ cup Greek yogurt

1 cup mixed berries

Instructions:

Mix rolled oats, mashed banana, eggs, baking powder, and honey to form a batter.

Heat a non-stick pan and cook pancakes until golden on each side.

Serve pancakes with Greek yogurt and mixed berries on top.

Nutritional Information (per serving):

Calories: 340

Protein: 14g

Carbs: 54g

Fat: 8g

Notes

_____

_____

_____

_____

_____

_____

Savory Veggie Omelette

Preparation Time:	**Cooking Time:**	**Servings:**
10 minutes	**10 minutes**	**2**

Ingredients:

4 eggs, whisked

1 cup spinach leaves, chopped

½ cup cherry tomatoes, halved

¼ cup feta cheese, crumbled

1 tbsp olive oil

Salt and pepper, to taste

Instructions:

Heat olive oil in a pan and sauté spinach leaves and cherry tomatoes until softened.

Pour whisked eggs over veggies and sprinkle feta cheese on top.

Cook omelette until eggs are set, fold in half and serve.

Nutritional Information (per serving):

Calories: 290

Protein: 18g

Carbs: 6g

Fat: 22g

Notes

_____

_____

_____

_____

_____

_____

Almond Butter and Banana Sandwich

Preparation Time:
5 minutes

Cooking Time:
0 minutes

Servings:
2

Ingredients:

4 slices whole-grain bread

2 tbsp almond butter, unsweetened

1 banana, sliced

1 tbsp honey

½ tsp cinnamon powder

Instructions:

Spread almond butter over two slices of bread.

Place banana slices on top, drizzle with honey, sprinkle with cinnamon, and top with the remaining slices of bread.

Serve immediately.

Nutritional Information (per serving):

Calories: 330

Protein: 11g

Carbs: 48g

Fat: 12g

Notes

_____

_____

_____

_____

_____

_____

Green Power Smoothie

Preparation Time:	Cooking Time:	Servings:
10 minutes	0 minutes	2

Ingredients:

1 cup kale leaves, chopped

1 cup pineapple chunks

1 banana

1 tbsp flaxseeds

1 cup coconut water

Instructions:

Blend kale leaves, pineapple chunks, banana, flaxseeds, and coconut water until smooth.

Pour the smoothie into glasses and serve immediately.

Nutritional Information (per serving):

Calories: 180

Protein: 3g

Carbs: 42g

Fat: 2g

Notes

_____

_____

_____

_____

_____

_____

Avocado Toast with Poached Eggs

Preparation Time:	Cooking Time:	Servings:
15 minutes	5 minutes	2

Ingredients:

2 slices whole-grain bread, toasted

1 avocado, mashed

2 eggs, poached

Salt and pepper, to taste

1 tbsp fresh parsley, chopped

Instructions:

Spread mashed avocado over toasted bread slices.

Place poached eggs on top, season with salt and pepper, and garnish with fresh parsley.

Serve immediately.

Nutritional Information (per serving):

Calories: 320

Protein: 14g

Carbs: 28g

Fat: 18g

Notes

_____

_____

_____

_____

_____

_____

Mango Coconut Smoothie

Preparation Time:

10 minutes

Cooking Time:

0 minutes

Servings:

2

Ingredients:

1 cup mango chunks

1 banana

1 cup coconut milk, unsweetened

1 tbsp chia seeds

Instructions:

Blend mango chunks, banana, coconut milk, and chia seeds until smooth.

Pour the smoothie into glasses and serve immediately.

Nutritional Information (per serving)

Calories: 240

Protein: 3g

Carbs: 36g

Fat: 10g

Notes

_____

_____

_____

_____

_____

_____

Berry Quinoa Breakfast Bowl

Preparation Time:	Cooking Time:	Servings:
10 minutes	0 minutes	2

Ingredients:

1 cup cooked quinoa

1 cup mixed berries (strawberries, blueberries, raspberries)

1 cup Greek yogurt

1 tbsp honey

2 tbsp almonds, sliced

Instructions:

Divide cooked quinoa between two bowls.

Top with mixed berries, Greek yogurt, honey, and sliced almonds.

Serve immediately.

Nutritional Information (per serving):

Calories: 340

Protein: 18g

Carbs: 50g

Fat: 8g

Notes

_____

_____

_____

_____

_____

_____

Fruity Chia Pudding

Preparation Time:	Cooking Time:	Servings:
10 minutes (+2 hours refrigeration)	0 minutes	2

Ingredients:

2 tbsp chia seeds

1 cup almond milk, unsweetened

1 cup mixed fruit (mango, kiwi, pineapple)

1 tbsp honey

1 tbsp coconut flakes, unsweetened

Instructions:

Mix chia seeds with almond milk and let sit in the refrigerator for at least 2 hours, or overnight.

Divide chia pudding between two bowls and top with mixed fruit, honey, and coconut flakes.

Nutritional Information (per serving):

Calories: 240

Protein: 5g

Carbs: 38g

Fat: 9g

Notes

_____

_____

_____

_____

_____

_____

Zesty Veggie Scramble

Preparation Time:	Cooking Time:	Servings:
10 minutes	10 minutes	2

Ingredients:

4 eggs, whisked

1 cup bell peppers, diced

1 tomato, diced

½ cup red onion, diced

1 tbsp olive oil

Salt and pepper, to taste

1 tbsp fresh cilantro, chopped

Instructions:

Sauté bell peppers, tomato, and red onion in olive oil until softened.

Pour whisked eggs over veggies and scramble until eggs are cooked.

Season with salt and pepper and garnish with fresh cilantro.

Nutritional Information (per serving):

Calories: 260

Protein: 14g

Carbs: 12g

Fat: 18g

Notes

_____

_____

_____

_____

_____

_____

Berry Nutty Oatmeal

Preparation Time:	**Cooking Time:**	**Servings:**
5 minutes	**10 minutes**	**2**

Ingredients:

1 cup rolled oats

2 cups water

1 cup mixed berries (strawberries, blueberries, raspberries)

2 tbsp almonds, chopped

1 tbsp honey

Instructions:

Cook rolled oats in water until tender.

Divide oatmeal between two bowls and top with mixed berries, chopped almonds, and honey.

Nutritional Information (per serving):

Calories: 270

Protein: 7g

Carbs: 45g

Fat: 8g

Notes

_____

_____

_____

_____

_____

_____

Protein-Packed Avocado Toast

Preparation Time:	Cooking Time:	Servings:
10 minutes	0 minutes	2

Ingredients:

2 slices whole-grain bread, toasted

1 avocado, mashed

4 slices turkey breast, nitrate-free

Salt and pepper, to taste

1 tbsp fresh parsley, chopped

Instructions:

Spread mashed avocado over toasted bread slices.

Place turkey slices on top, season with salt and pepper, and garnish with fresh parsley.

Serve immediately.

Nutritional Information (per serving):

Calories: 320

Protein: 20g

Carbs: 26g

Fat: 16g

Notes

_____

_____

_____

_____

_____

_____

Hearty Veggie Frittata

Preparation Time:	Cooking Time:	Servings:
10 minutes	0 minutes	2

Ingredients:

4 eggs, whisked

1 cup mixed veggies (zucchini, bell peppers, cherry tomatoes), diced

1 tbsp olive oil

Salt and pepper, to taste

1 tbsp fresh basil, chopped

Instructions:

Sauté mixed veggies in olive oil until tender.

Pour whisked eggs over veggies and cook until eggs are set.

Season with salt and pepper and garnish with fresh basil.

Nutritional Information (per serving):

Calories: 240

Protein: 14g

Carbs: 10g

Fat: 16g

Notes

_____

_____

_____

_____

_____

_____

Refreshing Cucumber Melon Smoothie

Preparation Time: **Cooking Time:**   **Servings:**

10 minutes   0 minutes   2

Ingredients:

1 cup cucumber, sliced   1 cup coconut water

1 cup honeydew melon, cubed   1 tbsp mint leaves

Instructions:

Blend cucumber, honeydew melon, coconut water, and mint leaves until smooth.
Pour the smoothie into glasses and serve immediately.

Nutritional Information (per serving):

Calories: 80   Carbs: 20g

Protein: 1g   Fat: 0g

Notes

_____

_____

_____

_____

_____

_____

Energizing Fruit and Nut Yogurt Parfait

Preparation Time:

10 minutes

Cooking Time:

0 minutes

Servings:

2

Ingredients:

1 cup Greek yogurt

1 cup mixed fruit (berries, kiwi, mango), diced

2 tbsp almonds, chopped

1 tbsp honey

Instructions:

Layer Greek yogurt, mixed fruit, chopped almonds, and honey in two glasses. Serve immediately.

Nutritional Information (per serving):

Calories: 270

Protein: 15g

Carbs: 34g

Fat: 10g

Notes

_____

_____

_____

_____

_____

_____

Savory Spinach and Mushroom Oatmeal

Preparation Time:

10 minutes

Cooking Time:

15 minutes

Servings:

2

Ingredients:

1 cup rolled oats

2 cups water

1 cup spinach leaves, chopped

1 cup mushrooms, sliced

1 tbsp olive oil

Salt and pepper, to taste

1 tbsp fresh parsley, chopped

Instructions:

Cook rolled oats in water until tender.

Sauté spinach leaves and mushrooms in olive oil until tender.

Mix veggies with cooked oatmeal, season with salt and pepper, and garnish with fresh parsley.

Nutritional Information (per serving):

Calories: 250

Protein: 7g

Carbs: 38g

Fat: 8g

Notes

_____

_____

_____

_____

_____

_____

Protein-Packed Quinoa Breakfast Bowl

Preparation Time:	Cooking Time:	Servings:
10 minutes	0 minutes	2

Ingredients:

1 cup cooked quinoa

1 cup Greek yogurt

1 cup mixed berries (strawberries, blueberries, raspberries)

1 tbsp honey

2 tbsp walnuts, chopped

Instructions:

Divide cooked quinoa between two bowls.

Top with Greek yogurt, mixed berries, honey, and chopped walnuts.

Serve immediately.

Nutritional Information (per serving):

Calories: 340	Carbs: 50g
Protein: 18g	Fat: 10g

Notes

_____

_____

_____

_____

_____

_____

5. Lunches to Love

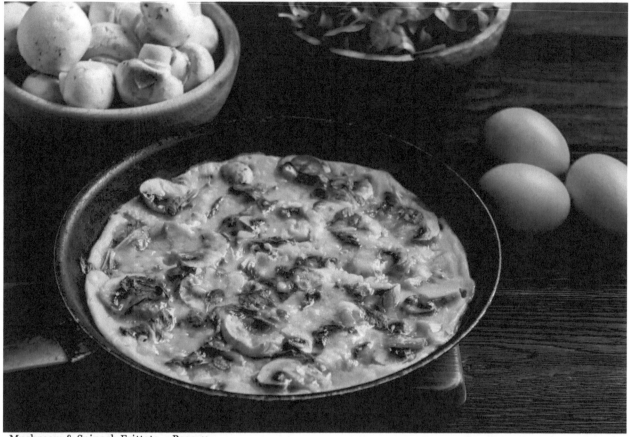

Mushroom & Spinach Frittata – Page 41

When the midday sun climbs high and stomachs begin to rumble, it's clear that lunchtime has arrived. In the world of clean eating, lunch is a pivotal moment to re-energize, refocus, and provide your body with the robust nourishment it needs to thrive through the remainder of the day. It's more than just a meal; it's an expression of love and respect for your body, served up on a plate.

Clean eating doesn't mean skimping on flavor; it's about letting the authentic tastes of high-quality ingredients shine. Each lunch recipe is a midday revitalization, a chance to refuel your body and rejoice in the natural simplicity of wholesome food. So, take this time to savor each bite, and let the energy of clean eating propel you through your day with clarity and vigor.

Herb-Crusted Chicken Salad

Preparation Time:	**Cooking Time:**	**Servings:**
15 minutes	**20 minutes**	**2**

Ingredients:

2 chicken breasts

2 tbsp olive oil

1 tbsp mixed herbs (thyme, rosemary, oregano)

4 cups mixed salad greens

1 cup cherry tomatoes, halved

1 cucumber, sliced

1 avocado, sliced

Salt and pepper, to taste

Instructions:

Preheat the oven to 400°F (200°C).

Rub chicken breasts with olive oil, mixed herbs, salt, and pepper.

Bake chicken for 20 minutes or until cooked through.

Arrange salad greens, tomatoes, cucumber, and avocado on plates.

Slice cooked chicken and place on top of the salad.

Drizzle with your favorite clean dressing and serve.

Nutritional Information (per serving):

Calories: 400

Protein: 35g

Carbs: 20g

Fat: 20g

Notes

_____

_____

_____

_____

_____

_____

Refreshing Cucumber Avocado Salad

Preparation Time:	Cooking Time:	Servings:
15 minutes	0 minutes	2

Ingredients:

2 cucumbers, sliced

1 avocado, diced

1 cup cherry tomatoes, halved

1 tbsp olive oil

1 tbsp lemon juice

Salt and pepper, to taste

Instructions:

In a bowl, combine cucumbers, avocado, and cherry tomatoes.

Drizzle with olive oil and lemon juice.

Season with salt and pepper.

Toss well and serve immediately.

Nutritional Information (per serving):

Calories: 270

Protein: 3g

Carbs: 20g

Fat: 22g

Notes

_____

_____

_____

_____

_____

_____

Spaghetti Squash with Tomato Basil Sauce

Preparation Time:	Cooking Time:	Servings:
10 minutes	45 minutes	2

Ingredients:

1 spaghetti squash, halved and seeds removed

2 cups fresh tomatoes, chopped

2 garlic cloves, minced

1 tbsp olive oil

1 tbsp fresh basil, chopped

Salt and pepper, to taste

Instructions:

Preheat the oven to 400°F (200°C).

Place spaghetti squash halves cut side down on a baking sheet.

Bake for 45 minutes or until squash is tender.

In a pan, heat olive oil and sauté garlic until golden.

Add tomatoes and simmer until sauce thickens.

Season with salt, pepper, and fresh basil.

Use a fork to scrape out the spaghetti squash strands.

Top with tomato basil sauce and serve.

Nutritional Information (per serving):

Calories: 200

Protein: 3g

Carbs: 40g

Fat: 7g

Notes

_____

_____

_____

_____

_____

_____

Zesty Lemon Tilapia

Preparation Time:	Cooking Time:	Servings:
10 minutes	15 minutes	2

Ingredients:

2 tilapia fillets

1 lemon, juiced

1 tbsp olive oil

2 tbsp fresh parsley, chopped

Salt and pepper, to taste

Instructions:

Preheat the oven to 375°F (190°C).

Place tilapia on a baking sheet and drizzle with olive oil and lemon juice.

Season with salt, pepper, and fresh parsley.

Bake for 15 minutes or until fish flakes easily with a fork.

Serve with a side of steamed vegetables or salad.

Nutritional Information (per serving):

Calories: 220

Protein: 35g

Carbs: 2g

Fat: 9g

Notes

_____

_____

_____

_____

_____

_____

Mushroom & Spinach Frittata

Preparation Time:	Cooking Time:	Servings:
10 minutes	15 minutes	2

Ingredients:

4 large eggs

1 cup fresh spinach, chopped

1 cup mushrooms, sliced

1 tbsp olive oil

Salt and pepper, to taste

2 tbsp fresh basil, chopped

Instructions:

Preheat oven to 375°F (190°C).

In a bowl, whisk eggs and season with salt and pepper.

Heat olive oil in an ovenproof skillet over medium heat.

Add mushrooms and sauté until tender.

Add spinach and cook until wilted.

Pour eggs over the vegetables and transfer the skillet to the oven.

Bake until the eggs are set, about 10 minutes. Garnish with fresh basil.

Nutritional Information (per serving):

Calories: 240

Protein: 16g

Carbs: 5g

Fat: 18g

Notes

_____

_____

_____

_____

_____

_____

Hearty Lentil Soup

Preparation Time: | **Cooking Time:** | **Servings:**
10 minutes | 40 minutes | 2

Ingredients:

1 cup dry lentils

1 onion, diced

2 carrots, sliced

2 celery stalks, sliced

2 garlic cloves, minced

1 can (14 oz) diced tomatoes

4 cups vegetable broth

2 tbsp olive oil

Salt and pepper, to taste

2 tbsp fresh parsley, chopped

Instructions:

Heat olive oil in a pot over medium heat.

Add onion, carrots, and celery and sauté until softened.

Stir in garlic until fragrant.

Add lentils, tomatoes, and vegetable broth.

Bring to a boil, then lower heat and simmer until lentils are tender.

Season with salt, pepper, and fresh parsley before serving.

Nutritional Information (per serving):

Calories: 350

Protein: 20g

Carbs: 45g

Fat: 10g

Notes

_____

_____

_____

_____

_____

_____

Spicy Pineapple Chicken

Preparation Time:	**Cooking Time:**	**Servings:**
15 minutes	**20 minutes**	**2**

Ingredients:

2 chicken breasts, cut into chunks

1 cup pineapple, diced

1 red bell pepper, sliced

1 tbsp olive oil

1 tbsp chili flakes

1 tbsp honey

Salt and pepper, to taste

Instructions:

Heat olive oil in a pan over medium heat.

Add chicken chunks and cook until browned and cooked through.

Add pineapple and bell pepper and sauté until tender.

Mix in chili flakes, honey, salt, and pepper.

Serve over cooked brown rice or quinoa.

Nutritional Information (per serving):

Calories: 410

Protein: 35g

Carbs: 40g

Fat: 10g

Notes

_____

_____

_____

_____

_____

_____

Grilled Veggie Platter

Preparation Time:
10 minutes

Cooking Time:
15 minutes

Servings:
2

Ingredients:

1 zucchini, sliced

1 yellow squash, sliced

1 red bell pepper, cut into chunks

1 cup cherry tomatoes

2 tbsp olive oil

Salt and pepper, to taste

2 tbsp balsamic glaze

Instructions:

Preheat the grill to medium-high heat.

Toss vegetables in olive oil, salt, and pepper.

Grill vegetables until slightly charred and tender.

Drizzle with balsamic glaze before serving.

Nutritional Information (per serving):

Calories: 260

Protein: 5g

Carbs: 25g

Fat: 18g

Notes

_____

_____

_____

_____

_____

_____

Baked Sweet Potato with Avocado Salsa

Preparation Time:	Cooking Time:	Servings:
10 minutes	45 minutes	2

Ingredients:

2 sweet potatoes

1 avocado, diced

1 cup cherry tomatoes, halved

1/4 cup red onion, diced

1 lime, juiced

2 tbsp fresh cilantro, chopped

Salt and pepper, to taste

Instructions:

Preheat the oven to 400°F (200°C).

Pierce sweet potatoes with a fork and bake for 45 minutes or until tender.

In a bowl, combine avocado, tomatoes, red onion, lime juice, cilantro, salt, and pepper.

Once sweet potatoes are done, split them open and top with avocado salsa.

Nutritional Information (per serving):

Calories: 320

Protein: 5g

Carbs: 50g

Fat: 15g

Notes

_____

_____

_____

_____

_____

_____

Spinach and Feta Stuffed Chicken

Preparation Time:	Cooking Time:	Servings:
10 minutes	25 minutes	2

Ingredients:

2 chicken breasts

1 cup fresh spinach, chopped

1/2 cup feta cheese, crumbled

1 tbsp olive oil

Salt and pepper, to taste

Instructions:

Preheat the oven to 375°F (190°C).

Cut a pocket into each chicken breast.

Stuff with spinach and feta cheese.

Seal with toothpicks and season with salt and pepper.

Heat olive oil in an ovenproof skillet and brown chicken on both sides.

Transfer skillet to the oven and bake until chicken is cooked through.

Nutritional Information (per serving):

Calories: 370	Carbs: 3g
Protein: 35g	Fat: 25g

Notes

_____

_____

_____

_____

_____

_____

Lemon Herb Quinoa Salad

Preparation Time:	Cooking Time:	Servings:
10 minutes	0 minutes	2

Ingredients:

1 cup cooked quinoa

1 cup mixed greens (spinach, arugula, etc.)

1/2 cucumber, diced

1/2 cup cherry tomatoes, halved

1/4 cup fresh parsley, chopped

1/4 cup fresh mint, chopped

1 lemon, juiced

2 tbsp olive oil

Salt and pepper, to taste

Instructions:

In a large bowl, combine cooked quinoa, mixed greens, cucumber, cherry tomatoes, parsley, and mint.

Drizzle with lemon juice and olive oil.

Toss well to combine and season with salt and pepper to taste before serving.

Nutritional Information (per serving):

Calories: 320	Carbs: 40g
Protein: 8g	Fat: 15g

Notes

_____
_____
_____
_____
_____
_____

Honey Mustard Grilled Salmon

Preparation Time:
10 minutes

Cooking Time:
15 minutes

Servings:
2

Ingredients:

2 salmon fillets

2 tbsp honey

2 tbsp Dijon mustard

1 tbsp olive oil

Salt and pepper, to taste

2 tbsp fresh chives, chopped

Instructions:

Preheat grill to medium heat.

In a bowl, mix honey, Dijon mustard, olive oil, salt, and pepper.

Brush salmon fillets with the honey mustard mixture.

Grill salmon for about 7 minutes on each side or until done.

Garnish with fresh chives before serving.

Nutritional Information (per serving):

Calories: 410

Protein: 35g

Carbs: 20g

Fat: 20g

Notes

_____

_____

_____

_____

_____

_____

Vegetable Stir-Fry with Brown Rice

Preparation Time:	Cooking Time:	Servings:
10 minutes	20 minutes	2

Ingredients:

1 cup mixed vegetables (broccoli, snap peas, carrots, etc.)

1 tbsp olive oil

2 tbsp soy sauce (low sodium)

1 tbsp sesame oil

1 cup cooked brown rice

Instructions:

Heat olive oil in a wok or large skillet over medium-high heat.

Add mixed vegetables and stir-fry until tender-crisp.

Drizzle with soy sauce and sesame oil and toss to coat.

Serve the vegetable stir-fry over cooked brown rice.

Nutritional Information (per serving):

Calories: 330

Protein: 6g

Carbs: 40g

Fat: 15g

Notes

_____

_____

_____

_____

_____

_____

Spaghetti Squash Primavera

Preparation Time:	**Cooking Time:**	**Servings:**
15 minutes	45 minutes	2

Ingredients:

1 spaghetti squash, halved and seeds removed

1 cup cherry tomatoes, halved

1/2 cup bell peppers, diced

1/2 cup zucchini, diced

2 tbsp olive oil

2 garlic cloves, minced

Salt and pepper, to taste

2 tbsp fresh basil, chopped

1/4 cup grated Parmesan cheese (optional)

Instructions:

Preheat the oven to 400°F (200°C).

Place spaghetti squash cut side down on a baking sheet and bake for about 35-40 minutes or until tender.

In a skillet, heat olive oil over medium heat.

Add garlic, tomatoes, bell peppers, and zucchini and sauté until soft.

Use a fork to scrape the strands of spaghetti squash into the skillet and toss with the vegetables.

Season with salt and pepper and garnish with fresh basil and Parmesan cheese if desired.

Nutritional Information (per serving):

Calories: 330

Protein: 9g

Carbs: 45g

Fat: 15g

Notes

_____

_____

_____

_____

_____

_____

Creamy Avocado and Spinach Pasta

Preparation Time:	Cooking Time:	Servings:
10 minutes	15 minutes	2

Ingredients:

2 servings of whole grain spaghetti or
pasta of choice

1 ripe avocado

2 cups fresh spinach

2 garlic cloves

2 tbsp lemon juice

2 tbsp olive oil

Salt and pepper to taste

Cherry tomatoes for garnish

Instructions:

Cook the pasta according to package instructions.

In a blender or food processor, combine avocado, spinach, garlic, lemon juice, olive oil, salt, and pepper. Blend until smooth.

Toss the cooked pasta with the avocado spinach sauce.

Serve garnished with cherry tomatoes.

Nutritional Information (per serving):

Calories: 420	Carbs: 60g
Protein: 12g	Fat: 18g

Notes

_____
_____
_____
_____
_____
_____

Apple Walnut Salad with Grilled Chicken

Preparation Time:	Cooking Time:	Servings:
10 minutes	15 minutes	2

Ingredients:

2 chicken breasts

2 cups mixed greens

1 apple, sliced

1/4 cup walnuts, chopped

1/4 cup feta cheese, crumbled (optional)

1 tbsp olive oil

1 tbsp balsamic vinegar

Salt and pepper, to taste

Instructions:

Season chicken breasts with salt and pepper and grill until fully cooked.

In a large bowl, combine mixed greens, apple slices, walnuts, and feta cheese.

Drizzle with olive oil and balsamic vinegar.

Toss the salad well and serve with grilled chicken on top.

Nutritional Information (per serving):

Calories: 410

Protein: 30g

Carbs: 20g

Fat: 25g

Notes

_____

_____

_____

_____

_____

_____

Spicy Avocado Tuna Salad

Preparation Time: **Cooking Time:**   **Servings:**

10 minutes   **0 minutes**   **2**

Ingredients:

1 can (150g) tuna in water, drained   2 tbsp fresh cilantro, chopped

1 ripe avocado, diced   1 lime, juiced

1/2 red onion, finely chopped   Salt and pepper, to taste

1 jalapeño, finely chopped

Instructions:

In a bowl, combine tuna, avocado, red onion, jalapeño, and cilantro.

Drizzle with lime juice and season with salt and pepper.

Toss well to combine before serving.

Nutritional Information (per serving):

Calories: 320   Carbs: 20g

Protein: 25g   Fat: 18g

Notes

_____

_____

_____

_____

_____

_____

Roasted Vegetable and Lentil Salad

Preparation Time:	Cooking Time:	Servings:
15 minutes	25 minutes	2

Ingredients:

1 cup cooked lentils

1 cup mixed vegetables (zucchini, cherry tomatoes, bell peppers), diced

2 tbsp olive oil

Salt and pepper, to taste

1 lemon, juiced

2 tbsp fresh parsley, chopped

Instructions:

Preheat the oven to 400°F (200°C).

Toss mixed vegetables with 1 tbsp olive oil and season with salt and pepper.

Roast vegetables in the oven until tender, about 20 minutes.

In a large bowl, combine roasted vegetables, cooked lentils, remaining olive oil, lemon juice, and fresh parsley.

Toss well to combine before serving.

Nutritional Information (per serving):

Calories: 350

Protein: 18g

Carbs: 40g

Fat: 15g

Notes

_____

_____

_____

_____

_____

_____

Herb-Infused Baked Salmon

Preparation Time:	Cooking Time:	Servings:
10 minutes	20 minutes	2

Ingredients:

2 salmon fillets

1 tbsp olive oil

1 tbsp fresh lemon juice

1 tbsp fresh dill, chopped

1 tbsp fresh parsley, chopped

Salt and pepper, to taste

1 lemon, sliced

Instructions:

Preheat oven to 375°F (190°C).

Place salmon fillets on a baking sheet.

Drizzle olive oil and lemon juice over the salmon.

Sprinkle with dill, parsley, salt, and pepper.

Place lemon slices on top of the salmon fillets.

Bake for 20 minutes or until salmon flakes easily with a fork.

Nutritional Information (per serving):

Calories: 340

Protein: 34g

Carbs: 3g

Fat: 21g

Notes

_____

_____

_____

_____

_____

_____

Ginger-Soy Infused Steamed Cod

Preparation Time:
10 minutes

Cooking Time:
15 minutes

Servings:
2

Ingredients:

2 Cod Fillets (200g each)

2 tbsp Low Sodium Soy Sauce

1 tbsp Freshly Grated Ginger

1 cup Mixed Steamed Vegetables
(Broccoli, Carrots, Snap Peas)

1 tbsp Olive Oil

1 tbsp Lemon Juice

Instructions:

Marinate cod fillets in soy sauce and ginger for 10 minutes.

Steam cod and vegetables until the fish is flaky and vegetables are tender.

Drizzle with olive oil and lemon juice before serving.

Nutritional Information (per serving):

Calories: 280

Protein: 32g

Carbs: 10g

Fat: 12g

Notes

_____

_____

_____

_____

_____

_____

Hearty Turkey and Vegetable Skillet

Preparation Time:	Cooking Time:	Servings:
10 minutes	20 minutes	2

Ingredients:

1/2 lb lean ground turkey

2 cups mixed vegetables (bell peppers, zucchini, cherry tomatoes), diced

1 tbsp olive oil

2 garlic cloves, minced

Salt and pepper, to taste

1 tbsp fresh basil, chopped

Instructions:

Heat olive oil in a skillet over medium heat.

Add garlic and sauté until golden.

Add ground turkey and cook until browned.

Add mixed vegetables, salt, and pepper.

Cook until vegetables are tender.

Garnish with fresh basil before serving.

Nutritional Information (per serving):

Calories: 330

Protein: 26g

Carbs: 20g

Fat: 16g

Notes

_____

_____

_____

_____

_____

_____

Spiced Quinoa and Vegetable Stir-Fry

Preparation Time:	Cooking Time:	Servings:
10 minutes	20 minutes	2

Ingredients:

1 cup cooked quinoa

2 cups mixed vegetables (carrots, snap peas, bell peppers), sliced

1 tbsp olive oil

2 tbsp low sodium soy sauce

1 tsp ground ginger

1 tsp garlic powder

1 tbsp fresh green onions, chopped

Instructions:

Heat olive oil in a wok or large skillet over medium-high heat.

Add mixed vegetables and stir-fry until tender-crisp.

Add cooked quinoa, soy sauce, ground ginger, and garlic powder to the wok.

Toss well to combine and garnish with green onions before serving.

Nutritional Information (per serving):

Calories: 330

Protein: 10g

Carbs: 50g

Fat: 10g

Notes

_____

_____

_____

_____

_____

_____

Sesame Ginger Chicken Salad

Preparation Time:
15 minutes

Cooking Time:
15 minutes

Servings:
2

Ingredients:

2 chicken breasts

2 cups mixed greens

1 cup mandarin orange segments

1/4 cup almonds, slivered

2 tbsp sesame oil

1 tbsp fresh ginger, grated

1 tbsp soy sauce (low sodium)

1 tbsp honey

Instructions:

Season chicken breasts with salt and pepper and grill until fully cooked.

In a large bowl, combine mixed greens, mandarin oranges, and almonds.

In a small bowl, whisk together sesame oil, ginger, soy sauce, and honey.

Drizzle dressing over the salad and toss well to combine.

Serve salad with sliced grilled chicken on top.

Nutritional Information (per serving):

Calories: 380

Protein: 30g

Carbs: 25g

Fat: 20g

Notes

_____

_____

_____

_____

_____

_____

Spicy Chickpea & Avocado Wrap

Preparation Time:	Cooking Time:	Servings:
10 minutes	10 minutes	2

Ingredients:

1 cup canned chickpeas, drained and rinsed

1 avocado, sliced

2 whole wheat wraps

1 cup fresh spinach leaves

1 tbsp olive oil

1 tsp chili flakes

Salt and pepper, to taste

Instructions:

Heat olive oil in a skillet over medium heat.

Add chickpeas, chili flakes, salt, and pepper.

Sauté until chickpeas are golden and crispy.

Arrange chickpeas, avocado slices, and fresh spinach leaves on the wraps.

Roll up the wraps and serve immediately.

Nutritional Information (per serving):

Calories: 410	Carbs: 45g
Protein: 12g	Fat: 22g

Notes

_____

_____

_____

_____

_____

_____

Grilled Eggplant and Tomato Stacks

Preparation Time:	Cooking Time:	Servings:
10 minutes	15 minutes	2

Ingredients:

1 large eggplant, sliced into rounds

2 large tomatoes, sliced

1/4 cup fresh basil leaves

2 tbsp olive oil

2 tbsp balsamic glaze

Salt and pepper to taste

Instructions:

Preheat grill to medium-high heat.

Brush eggplant slices with olive oil and season with salt and pepper.

Grill eggplant for 3-4 minutes on each side or until tender.

Stack grilled eggplant with tomato slices and fresh basil.

Drizzle with balsamic glaze before serving.

Nutritional Information (per serving):

Calories: 180

Protein: 3g

Carbs: 20g

Fat: 10g

Notes

_____

_____

_____

_____

_____

_____

Garlic & Herb Roasted Chicken and Veggies

Preparation Time: **Cooking Time:**   **Servings:**

15 minutes   **25 minutes**   **2**

Ingredients:

2 chicken breasts

2 cups mixed vegetables (carrots, broccoli, bell peppers), chopped

2 tbsp olive oil

2 garlic cloves, minced

1 tbsp mixed herbs (rosemary, thyme, oregano)

Salt and pepper, to taste

Instructions:

Preheat oven to 400°F (200°C).

Toss chicken and vegetables with olive oil, garlic, herbs, salt, and pepper.

Arrange on a baking sheet in a single layer.

Roast until chicken is cooked through and vegetables are tender, about 25 minutes.

Nutritional Information (per serving):

Calories: 360   Carbs: 20g

Protein: 30g   Fat: 18g

Notes

_____

_____

_____

_____

_____

_____

6. Dinners to Savor

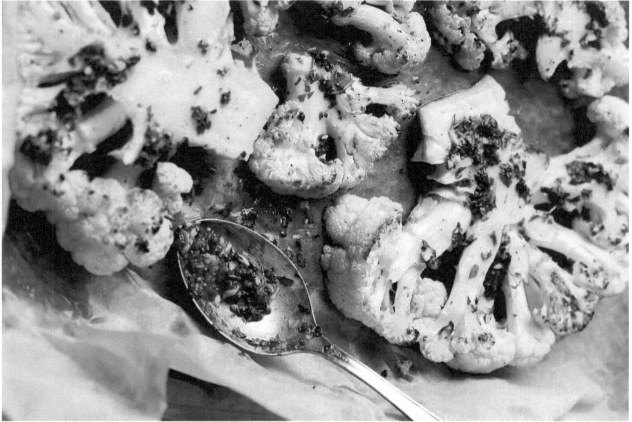

Cauliflower Steak with Chimichurri Sauce – Page 69

Dinner is a tranquil time, a moment to unwind after the day's hustle and bustle, and in the realm of clean eating, it's an opportunity to nourish your body with pure, whole foods that satisfy and comfort without heaviness or regret.

Dinner in clean eating is about balance, simplicity, and returning to the roots of culinary enjoyment. It's the last savory note of your day, a melody of nutrient-rich, unprocessed foods that nurture your body, promote restful sleep, and prepare you for the adventures of tomorrow.

Herb-Crusted Chicken with Sweet Potato Mash

Preparation Time:	Cooking Time:	Servings:
10 minutes	**25 minutes**	**2**

Ingredients:

2 Chicken Breasts (200g each)

2 tbsp Mixed Fresh Herbs (Thyme, Rosemary, Parsley), chopped

2 Sweet Potatoes, peeled and diced

1 tbsp Olive Oil

Salt and Pepper to taste

1 tbsp Lemon Juice

Instructions:

Preheat oven to 375°F (190°C).

Coat chicken breasts with herbs, olive oil, salt, and pepper.

Bake until the internal temperature reaches 165°F (74°C), about 20 minutes.

Boil sweet potatoes until tender, mash and season with salt, and pepper.

Serve chicken with sweet potato mash and a drizzle of lemon juice.

Nutritional Information (per serving):

Calories: 390

Protein: 30g

Carbs: 30g

Fat: 16g

Notes

_____

_____

_____

_____

_____

_____

Lemon-Herb Tilapia with Asparagus

Preparation Time:	**Cooking Time:**	**Servings:**
5 minutes	**15 minutes**	**2**

Ingredients:

2 Tilapia Fillets (150g each)

1 bunch Asparagus, trimmed

2 tbsp Olive Oil

1 Lemon, sliced

2 tbsp Fresh Parsley, chopped

Salt and Pepper to taste

Instructions:

Preheat oven to 400°F (200°C).

Arrange tilapia, asparagus, and lemon slices on a baking sheet.

Drizzle with olive oil and season with salt and pepper.

Bake until fish is flaky and asparagus is tender, about 15 minutes.

Garnish with fresh parsley before serving.

Nutritional Information (per serving):

Calories: 280

Protein: 28g

Carbs: 8g

Fat: 16g

Notes

_____

_____

_____

_____

_____

_____

Herb-Crusted Tilapia with Quinoa

Preparation Time:
10 minutes

Cooking Time:
15 minutes

Servings:
2

Ingredients:

2 Tilapia Fillets (150g each)

1 cup Cooked Quinoa

1 tbsp Olive Oil

1 tbsp Mixed Fresh Herbs (Parsley, Thyme, Dill), finely chopped

Salt and Pepper to taste

1 Lemon, sliced

Instructions:

Preheat oven to 400°F (200°C).

Season tilapia fillets with olive oil, herbs, salt, and pepper.

Place on a baking sheet and arrange lemon slices on top.

Bake until fish flakes easily with a fork, about 15 minutes.

Serve over cooked quinoa.

Nutritional Information (per serving):

Calories: 320

Protein: 28g

Carbs: 25g

Fat: 10g

Notes

_____

_____

_____

_____

_____

_____

Mushroom and Spinach Stuffed Chicken Breast

Preparation Time:	Cooking Time:	Servings:
15 minutes	25 minutes	2

Ingredients:

2 Chicken Breasts (200g each)

1 cup Sliced Mushrooms

1 cup Fresh Spinach, chopped

2 tbsp Olive Oil

Salt and Pepper to taste

1 tbsp Fresh Lemon Juice

Instructions:

Preheat oven to 375°F (190°C).

Sauté mushrooms and spinach in 1 tbsp olive oil until tender. Set aside.

Create a pocket in each chicken breast and stuff with mushroom-spinach mixture.

Secure with toothpicks and season with salt, pepper, and remaining olive oil.

Bake until internal temperature reaches 165°F (74°C), about 25 minutes.

Drizzle with fresh lemon juice before serving.

Nutritional Information (per serving):

Calories: 320

Protein: 30g

Carbs: 5g

Fat: 20g

Notes

_____

_____

_____

_____

_____

_____

Spicy Radish Tacos

Preparation Time:	Cooking Time:	Servings:
15 minutes	**10 minutes**	**2**

Ingredients:

1 cup radishes, thinly sliced	4 corn tortillas
1 tbsp olive oil	1/2 cup black beans, cooked
1 tsp chili powder	1/4 cup plain Greek yogurt
1/2 tsp cumin	Fresh cilantro, for garnish
1/4 tsp garlic powder	Lime wedges, for serving

Instructions:

In a skillet, heat olive oil over medium heat. Add radishes, chili powder, cumin, and garlic powder. Cook for 5-7 minutes or until radishes are tender.

Warm tortillas according to package instructions.

Assemble tacos by layering black beans, spicy radishes, and a dollop of Greek yogurt on each tortilla.

Garnish with fresh cilantro and serve with lime wedges.

Nutritional Value (per serving):

Calories: 320	Carbs: 50g
Protein: 12g	Fat: 9g

Notes

_____
_____
_____
_____
_____
_____

Cauliflower Steak with Chimichurri Sauce

Preparation Time:	Cooking Time:	Servings:
15 minutes	20 minutes	2

Ingredients:

1 large cauliflower head, sliced into 1-inch thick "steaks"

2 tbsp olive oil

Salt and pepper to taste

Homemade Chimichurri Sauce:

- 1 cup fresh parsley, finely chopped

- 1/2 cup fresh cilantro, finely chopped

- 2 garlic cloves, minced

- 1/4 cup olive oil

- 2 tbsp red wine vinegar

- 1/4 tsp red pepper flakes

- Salt and pepper to taste

Instructions:

Preheat oven to 400°F (200°C).

Brush both sides of cauliflower steaks with olive oil and season with salt and pepper.

Place on a baking sheet and roast for 20 minutes, flipping halfway through.

For the chimichurri sauce, combine all ingredients in a bowl and mix well.

Serve cauliflower steaks drizzled with chimichurri sauce.

Nutritional Information (per serving):

Calories: 250

Protein: 5g

Carbs: 15g

Fat: 20g

Notes

_____

_____

_____

_____

_____

_____

Grilled Salmon with Avocado Salsa

Preparation Time: | **Cooking Time:** | **Servings:**
10 minutes | 10 minutes | 2

Ingredients:

2 Salmon Fillets (150g each) | Salt and Pepper to taste
1 Avocado, diced | 1 tbsp Olive Oil
1 Tomato, diced | 1 tbsp Fresh Cilantro, chopped
1 tbsp Fresh Lime Juice

Instructions:

Preheat grill to medium-high heat.

Season salmon with salt, pepper, and olive oil.

Grill salmon for about 5 minutes per side or until desired doneness.

In a bowl, mix avocado, tomato, lime juice, cilantro, salt, and pepper.

Top grilled salmon with avocado salsa before serving.

Nutritional Information (per serving):

Calories: 410 | Carbs: 12g
Protein: 25g | Fat: 30g

Notes

_____
_____
_____
_____
_____
_____

Sweet and Spicy Baked Pineapple Chicken

Preparation Time:	Cooking Time:	Servings:
10 minutes	20 minutes	2

Ingredients:

2 Chicken Breasts (200g each)

1 cup Pineapple Chunks

1 tbsp Honey

1 tbsp Sriracha Sauce

1 tbsp Olive Oil

Salt and Pepper to taste

Instructions:

Preheat oven to 375°F (190°C).

Mix honey and Sriracha sauce and marinate chicken breasts in the mixture for 10 minutes.

Heat olive oil in a skillet and sear chicken on both sides until golden, about 3 minutes per side.

Add pineapple chunks to the skillet and transfer to the oven.

Bake until chicken is cooked through, about 15 minutes.

Nutritional Information (per serving):

Calories: 350

Protein: 30g

Carbs: 30g

Fat: 12g

Notes

_____

_____

_____

_____

_____

_____

Roasted Beet and Goat Cheese Salad

Preparation Time:	Cooking Time:	Servings:
10 minutes	45 minutes	2

Ingredients:

2 medium-sized beets, peeled and diced

2 cups mixed salad greens (like arugula, spinach, and romaine)

1/4 cup goat cheese, crumbled

1/4 cup walnuts, toasted

2 tbsp olive oil

1 tbsp balsamic vinegar

Salt and pepper to taste

Instructions:

Preheat oven to 400°F (200°C).

Toss beets in 1 tbsp olive oil, salt, and pepper. Spread on a baking sheet.

Roast beets for 40-45 minutes or until tender.

In a large bowl, combine salad greens, roasted beets, goat cheese, and walnuts.

Drizzle with remaining olive oil and balsamic vinegar. Toss to combine.

Nutritional Information (per serving):

Calories: 280

Protein: 8g

Carbs: 20g

Fat: 20g

Notes

_____

_____

_____

_____

_____

_____

Cajun Spiced Sweet Potato Fries

Preparation Time:	Cooking Time:	Servings:
10 minutes	30 minutes	2

Ingredients:

2 Sweet Potatoes, cut into fries

1 tbsp Olive Oil

1 tbsp Cajun Spice Mix

Salt to taste

2 tbsp Greek Yogurt (for dipping)

Instructions:

Preheat oven to 425°F (220°C).

Toss sweet potato fries with olive oil, Cajun spice, and salt.

Arrange on a baking sheet in a single layer.

Bake until crispy and golden, about 30 minutes, turning halfway through.

Serve with Greek yogurt on the side.

Nutritional Information (per serving):

Calories: 290

Protein: 5g

Carbs: 45g

Fat: 10g

Notes

_____

_____

_____

_____

_____

_____

Mango Avocado Salsa Chicken

Preparation Time:	Cooking Time:	Servings:
15 minutes	**20 minutes**	**2**

Ingredients:

2 Chicken Breasts (200g each)

1 Mango, diced

1 Avocado, diced

1 tbsp Fresh Lime Juice

Salt and Pepper to taste

1 tbsp Olive Oil

1 tbsp Fresh Cilantro, chopped

Instructions:

Preheat grill to medium-high heat.

Season chicken with salt, pepper, and olive oil.

Grill chicken for about 6-7 minutes per side or until internal temperature reaches 165°F (74°C).

In a bowl, mix mango, avocado, lime juice, cilantro, salt, and pepper.

Serve grilled chicken topped with mango avocado salsa.

Nutritional Information (per serving):

Calories: 410

Protein: 30g

Carbs: 25g

Fat: 22g

Notes

_____

_____

_____

_____

_____

_____

Zesty Lemon Asparagus Shrimp

Preparation Time:	Cooking Time:	Servings:
10 minutes	15 minutes	2

Ingredients:

2 cups Fresh Asparagus, trimmed and cut into pieces

200g Shrimp, peeled and deveined

1 tbsp Olive Oil

Salt and Pepper to taste

1 tbsp Fresh Lemon Zest

1 tbsp Fresh Lemon Juice

Instructions:

Heat olive oil in a skillet over medium-high heat.

Add shrimp and asparagus, season with salt and pepper.

Cook until shrimp is pink and asparagus is tender-crisp, about 5-7 minutes.

Stir in lemon zest and lemon juice before serving.

Nutritional Information (per serving):

Calories: 220

Protein: 25g

Carbs: 10g

Fat: 10g

Notes

_____

_____

_____

_____

_____

_____

Butternut Squash and Spinach Risotto

Preparation Time:

15 minutes

Cooking Time:

30 minutes

Servings:

2

Ingredients:

1 cup arborio rice

2 cups butternut squash, cubed

2 cups fresh spinach

1 onion, finely chopped

2 garlic cloves, minced

4 cups vegetable broth

2 tbsp olive oil

Salt and pepper to taste

Grated parmesan for garnish

Instructions:

In a large skillet, heat olive oil over medium heat. Add onion and garlic and sauté until translucent.

Add arborio rice and stir for 2 minutes.

Gradually add vegetable broth, one cup at a time, stirring constantly until the liquid is absorbed.

When the rice is almost cooked, add butternut squash and continue cooking until the squash is tender.

Stir in spinach and cook until wilted.

Season with salt and pepper and garnish with grated parmesan.

Nutritional Information (per serving):

Calories: 420

Protein: 10g

Carbs: 75g

Fat: 10g

Notes

_____

_____

_____

_____

_____

_____

Mediterranean Chickpea Salad

Preparation Time:	Cooking Time:	Servings:
10 minutes	0 minutes	2

Ingredients:

1 cup Cooked Chickpeas

1 cup Mixed Vegetables (cucumber, cherry tomatoes, red onion), diced

1 tbsp Olive Oil

1 tbsp Fresh Lemon Juice

Salt and Pepper to taste

1 tbsp Fresh Parsley, chopped

Instructions:

In a bowl, mix chickpeas, mixed vegetables, olive oil, lemon juice, salt, and pepper. Garnish with fresh parsley before serving.

Nutritional Information (per serving):

Calories: 260

Protein: 9g

Carbs: 35g

Fat: 10g

Notes

_____

_____

_____

_____

_____

_____

Balsamic Glazed Salmon

Preparation Time:	Cooking Time:	Servings:
10 minutes	15 minutes	2

Ingredients:

2 Salmon Fillets (150g each)
2 tbsp Balsamic Vinegar
1 tbsp Olive Oil

1 tbsp Honey
Salt and Pepper to taste
1 tbsp Fresh Basil, chopped

Instructions:

Preheat oven to 400°F (200°C).

In a bowl, mix balsamic vinegar, olive oil, honey, salt, and pepper.

Place salmon on a baking sheet and brush with balsamic mixture.

Bake for 15 minutes or until salmon flakes easily with a fork.

Garnish with fresh basil before serving.

Nutritional Information (per serving):

Calories: 320
Protein: 25g

Carbs: 15g
Fat: 17g

Notes

_____
_____
_____
_____
_____
_____

Stuffed Bell Peppers

Preparation Time:	Cooking Time:	Servings:
15 minutes	**25 minutes**	**2**

Ingredients:

2 Bell Peppers, halved and seeds removed

1 cup Cooked Brown Rice

1 cup Black Beans, cooked

1 cup Corn Kernels, cooked

1 tbsp Olive Oil

Salt and Pepper to taste

1 tbsp Fresh Cilantro, chopped

Instructions:

Preheat oven to 375°F (190°C).

In a bowl, mix brown rice, black beans, corn, olive oil, salt, and pepper.

Stuff bell pepper halves with the mixture and place on a baking sheet.

Bake for 25 minutes or until peppers are tender.

Garnish with fresh cilantro before serving.

Nutritional Information (per serving):

Calories: 380

Protein: 10g

Carbs: 65g

Fat: 9g

Notes

_____

_____

_____

_____

_____

_____

Roasted Vegetable Medley

Preparation Time:	Cooking Time:	Servings:
10 minutes	20 minutes	2

Ingredients:

1 cup Mixed Vegetables (zucchini, cherry tomatoes, bell peppers), chopped

1 tbsp Olive Oil

Salt and Pepper to taste

1 tbsp Fresh Basil, chopped

Instructions:

Preheat oven to 400°F (200°C).

Toss vegetables in olive oil, salt, and pepper.

Spread on a baking sheet and roast for 20 minutes or until vegetables are tender.

Garnish with fresh basil before serving.

Nutritional Information (per serving):

Calories: 120

Protein: 3g

Carbs: 10g

Fat: 8g

Notes

_____

_____

_____

_____

_____

_____

Pomegranate Roasted Brussels Sprouts

Preparation Time:	Cooking Time:	Servings:
10 minutes	**25 minutes**	**2**

Ingredients:

2 cups Brussels sprouts, halved

2 tbsp olive oil

Salt and pepper, to taste

1/2 cup pomegranate arils

1 tbsp balsamic glaze

Instructions:

Preheat the oven to 400°F (200°C).

Toss Brussels sprouts with olive oil, salt, and pepper on a baking sheet.

Roast for 20-25 minutes or until tender and caramelized.

Toss roasted Brussels sprouts with pomegranate arils and drizzle with balsamic glaze.

Serve immediately.

Nutritional Value (per serving):

Calories: 250

Protein: 8g

Carbs: 30g

Fat: 14g

Notes

_____

_____

_____

_____

_____

_____

Grilled Lemon Herb Chicken

Preparation Time:	Cooking Time:	Servings:
10 minutes	20 minutes	2

Ingredients:

2 Chicken Breasts (150g each)
1 tbsp Olive Oil
1 tbsp Fresh Lemon Juice

1 tbsp Fresh Thyme, chopped
Salt and Pepper to taste
1 tbsp Fresh Parsley, chopped

Instructions:

Preheat grill to medium-high heat.

Mix olive oil, lemon juice, thyme, salt, and pepper and marinate chicken for at least 30 minutes.

Grill chicken for about 7 minutes per side or until the internal temperature reaches 165°F (74°C).

Garnish with fresh parsley before serving.

Nutritional Information (per serving):

Calories: 300	Carbs: 3g
Protein: 27g	Fat: 19g

Notes

_____
_____
_____
_____
_____
_____

Sweet Potato and Black Bean Bowl

Preparation Time: **Cooking Time:**   **Servings:**

10 minutes   **20 minutes**   **2**

Ingredients:

1 Sweet Potato, diced   1 tbsp Olive Oil

1 cup Black Beans, cooked   Salt and Pepper to taste

1 cup Quinoa, cooked   1 tbsp Fresh Cilantro, chopped

Instructions:

Sauté sweet potato in olive oil until tender.

Mix with black beans and quinoa, season with salt and pepper.

Garnish with fresh cilantro before serving.

Nutritional Information (per serving):

Calories: 360   Carbs: 60g

Protein: 14g   Fat: 8g

Notes

_____

_____

_____

_____

_____

_____

Butternut Squash and Kale Risotto

Preparation Time:	Cooking Time:	Servings:
10 minutes	30 minutes	2

Ingredients:

1 cup arborio rice

2 cups vegetable broth

1 cup butternut squash, diced

1 cup kale, chopped

1/4 cup Parmesan cheese, grated

1 garlic clove, minced

1 tbsp olive oil

Salt and pepper to taste

Instructions:

In a pot, heat olive oil over medium heat. Add garlic and sauté for 1 minute.

Add rice and stir to coat with oil.

Gradually add vegetable broth, 1/2 cup at a time, stirring constantly until liquid is absorbed.

When rice is almost cooked, stir in butternut squash and kale.

Continue cooking until rice is tender and creamy.

Stir in Parmesan cheese and season with salt and pepper.

Nutritional Information (per serving):

Calories: 400

Protein: 10g

Carbs: 70g

Fat: 10g

Notes

_____

_____

_____

_____

_____

_____

Herb-Crusted Salmon

Preparation Time:	Cooking Time:	Servings:
10 minutes	**15 minutes**	**2**

Ingredients:

2 Salmon Fillets (150g each)

1 tbsp Olive Oil

1 tbsp Mixed Herbs (dill, parsley, chives), chopped

Salt and Pepper to taste

Lemon wedges for serving

Instructions:

Preheat the oven to 375°F (190°C).

Place salmon on a baking sheet and brush with olive oil.

Sprinkle herbs, salt, and pepper over salmon.

Bake for 15 minutes or until salmon flakes easily with a fork.

Serve with lemon wedges.

Nutritional Information (per serving):

Calories: 320

Protein: 34g

Carbs: 1g

Fat: 20g

Notes

_____

_____

_____

_____

_____

_____

Veggie-Packed Stir Fry

Preparation Time:

15 minutes

Cooking Time:

10 minutes

Servings:

2

Ingredients:

1 cup Mixed Vegetables (broccoli, bell peppers, snap peas, carrots), chopped

1 tbsp Olive Oil

1 tbsp Low-Sodium Soy Sauce

1 tbsp Fresh Ginger, grated

1 tbsp Fresh Cilantro, chopped

Instructions:

Heat oil in a pan over medium heat.

Add vegetables and stir-fry until tender, about 7-8 minutes.

Mix in soy sauce and ginger and stir well.

Garnish with fresh cilantro before serving.

Nutritional Information (per serving):

Calories: 150

Protein: 5g

Carbs: 20g

Fat: 7g

Notes

_____

_____

_____

_____

_____

_____

Grilled Portobello Mushrooms with Quinoa Salad

Preparation Time:	Cooking Time:	Servings:
15 minutes	**15 minutes**	**2**

Ingredients:

2 large portobello mushrooms

1 cup cooked quinoa

1/4 cup cherry tomatoes, halved

1/4 cup cucumber, diced

2 tbsp feta cheese, crumbled

2 tbsp olive oil

1 tbsp balsamic vinegar

Salt and pepper to taste

Instructions:

Preheat grill to medium-high heat.

Brush portobello mushrooms with olive oil and season with salt and pepper.

Grill mushrooms for 5-7 minutes on each side or until tender.

In a bowl, mix quinoa, cherry tomatoes, cucumber, feta, balsamic vinegar, salt, and pepper.

Serve grilled mushrooms topped with quinoa salad.

Nutritional Information (per serving):

Calories: 320

Protein: 10g

Carbs: 35g

Fat: 15g

Notes

_____

_____

_____

_____

_____

_____

Lemon Herb Grilled Shrimp

Preparation Time:	Cooking Time:	Servings:
10 minutes	10 minutes	2

Ingredients:

20 large shrimp, peeled and deveined

2 tbsp olive oil

Juice of 1 lemon

1 tbsp fresh parsley, chopped

1 tbsp fresh dill, chopped

Salt and pepper to taste

Instructions:

In a bowl, mix olive oil, lemon juice, parsley, dill, salt, and pepper.

Add shrimp and marinate for 10 minutes.

Preheat grill to medium-high heat.

Grill shrimp for 2-3 minutes on each side or until pink and opaque.

Serve with a side of steamed vegetables or salad.

Nutritional Information (per serving):

Calories: 200

Protein: 25g

Carbs: 2g

Fat: 10g

Notes

_____

_____

_____

_____

_____

_____

Spicy Bean Soup

Preparation Time:	Cooking Time:	Servings:
10 minutes	**20 minutes**	**2**

Ingredients:

1 cup Mixed Beans, cooked (black beans, kidney beans, white beans)

1 cup Vegetable Broth

1 tbsp Olive Oil

1 tsp Chili Powder

Salt and Pepper to taste

1 tbsp Fresh Cilantro, chopped

Instructions:

Heat oil in a pot over medium heat.

Add beans, broth, chili powder, salt, and pepper.

Bring to a boil, then reduce heat and simmer for 20 minutes.

Garnish with fresh cilantro before serving.

Nutritional Information (per serving):

Calories: 240

Protein: 14g

Carbs: 35g

Fat: 7g

Notes

_____

_____

_____

_____

_____

_____

7. Snacks to Relish

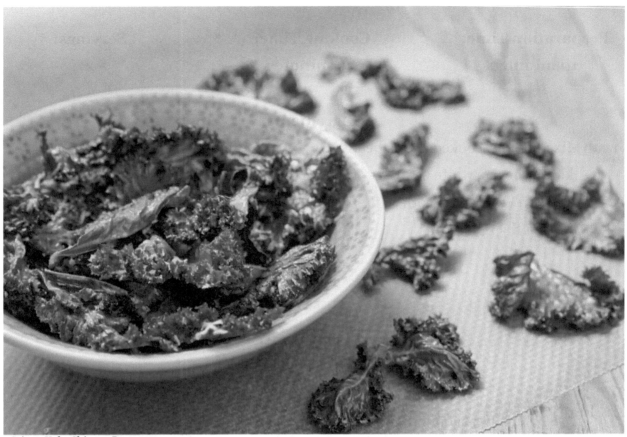

Crispy Kale Chips – Page 94

In the world of clean eating, snacks are not just a mindless munching affair; they're purposeful mini-meals that energize, satisfy, and provide essential nutrients between your main meals. It's a delightful morsel that satiates sweet cravings while providing nourishing energy.

Clean eating snacks are about conscious indulgence, enjoying foods that are as close to their natural state as possible, and listening to your body's needs. They're little parcels of nourishment that make healthy living a joyful journey.

Carrot and Cucumber Sticks with Hummus

Preparation Time:	Cooking Time:	Servings:
10 minutes	0 minutes	2

Ingredients:

1 large Carrot, peeled and cut into sticks

1 medium Cucumber, cut into sticks

½ cup Homemade Hummus

Homemade Hummus:

- 1 cup canned chickpeas, drained and rinsed
- 1 tbsp tahini
- 1 clove garlic, minced
- Zest and juice of 1 small lemon
- 1 tbsp Olive Oil
- 1 tbsp Mixed Fresh Herbs
- Salt and Pepper to taste
- 1-2 tbsp cold water

Instructions:

Arrange carrot and cucumber sticks on a plate.

For the homemade hummus, combine all ingredients in a blender or food processor and blend until smooth. If the mixture is too thick, add cold water, one tablespoon at a time, until you reach the desired consistency.

Serve carrot and cucumber sticks with homemade hummus.

Nutritional Information (per serving):

Calories: 150	Carbs: 20g
Protein: 5g	Fat: 7g

Notes

_____

_____

_____

_____

_____

_____

Roasted Sweet Potato Wedges

Preparation Time:	Cooking Time:	Servings:
10 minutes	30 minutes	2

Ingredients:

1 large Sweet Potato, washed and cut into wedges

1 tbsp Olive Oil

Salt and Pepper to taste

½ tsp Paprika

Instructions:

Preheat oven to 400°F (200°C).

Toss sweet potato wedges with olive oil, salt, pepper, and paprika.

Spread on a baking sheet in a single layer.

Bake until tender and golden brown, about 30 minutes, turning once.

Nutritional Information (per serving):

Calories: 180

Protein: 2g

Carbs: 32g

Fat: 7g

Notes

_____

_____

_____

_____

_____

_____

Zucchini and Corn Sauté

Preparation Time:
10 minutes

Cooking Time:
10 minutes

Servings:
2

Ingredients:

1 medium Zucchini, diced

½ cup Corn Kernels, fresh or frozen

1 tbsp Olive Oil

Salt and Pepper to taste

1 tbsp Fresh Parsley, chopped

Instructions:

Heat oil in a pan over medium heat.

Add zucchini and corn, season with salt and pepper.

Sauté until vegetables are tender, about 10 minutes.

Garnish with fresh parsley before serving.

Nutritional Information (per serving):

Calories: 130

Protein: 3g

Carbs: 17g

Fat: 7g

Notes

_____

_____

_____

_____

_____

_____

Crispy Kale Chips

Preparation Time:	Cooking Time:	Servings:
10 minutes	20 minutes	2

Ingredients:

1 bunch of Kale, washed and dried   Salt to taste

1 tbsp Olive Oil

Instructions:

Preheat oven to 350°F (180°C).

Tear kale into bite-sized pieces, removing any thick stems.

Toss kale in olive oil and sprinkle with salt.

Spread on a baking sheet in a single layer.

Bake until crisp but not browned, about 15-20 minutes, stirring halfway through.

Nutritional Information (per serving):

Calories: 100   Carbs: 7g

Protein: 2g   Fat: 7g

Notes

_____

_____

_____

_____

_____

_____

Cherry Tomato and Mozzarella Salad

Preparation Time:	Cooking Time:	Servings:
10 minutes	0 minutes	2

Ingredients:

1 cup Cherry Tomatoes, halved

½ cup Mozzarella Balls

1 tbsp Olive Oil

Salt and Pepper to taste

1 tbsp Fresh Basil, chopped

Instructions:

Mix tomatoes and mozzarella in a bowl.

Drizzle with olive oil, season with salt and pepper.

Garnish with fresh basil before serving.

Nutritional Information (per serving):

Calories: 170

Protein: 8g

Carbs: 5g

Fat: 14g

Notes

_____

_____

_____

_____

_____

_____

Mixed Nuts and Seeds

Preparation Time:	Cooking Time:	Servings:
2 minutes	0 minutes	2

Ingredients:

½ cup Mixed Nuts (almonds, walnuts, pecans)

¼ cup Mixed Seeds (pumpkin, sunflower)

Instructions:

Mix nuts and seeds in a bowl.

Serve as a nutritious and satisfying snack.

Nutritional Information (per serving):

Calories: 330

Carbs: 12g

Protein: 10g

Fat: 30g

Notes

_____

_____

_____

_____

_____

_____

Baked Radish Chips

Preparation Time:
10 minutes

Cooking Time:
10 minutes

Servings:
2

Ingredients:

2 cups radishes, thinly sliced

1 tbsp olive oil

1/2 tsp paprika

Salt, to taste

Instructions:

Preheat the oven to 375°F (190°C). Line a baking sheet with parchment paper.

Toss radish slices with olive oil, paprika, and salt.

Arrange radish slices in a single layer on the baking sheet.

Bake for 10-12 minutes or until crisp and golden.

Allow to cool before serving.

Nutritional Value (per serving):

Calories: 90

Protein: 1g

Carbs: 5g

Fat: 7g

Notes

_____

_____

_____

_____

_____

_____

Oven-Roasted Brussel Sprouts

Preparation Time:
10 minutes

Cooking Time:
20 minutes

Servings:
2

Ingredients:

2 cups Brussel Sprouts, washed and halved

1 tbsp Olive Oil

Salt and Pepper to taste

Instructions:

Preheat oven to 400°F (200°C).

Toss brussel sprouts with olive oil, salt, and pepper.

Spread on a baking sheet in a single layer.

Roast until golden and crispy, about 20 minutes, stirring once.

Nutritional Information (per serving):

Calories: 120

Carbs: 10g

Protein: 4g

Fat: 8g

Notes

_____

_____

_____

_____

_____

_____

Quinoa and Vegetable Salad

Preparation Time:	Cooking Time:	Servings:
10 minutes	0 minutes	2

Ingredients:

1 cup Quinoa, cooked

1 cup Mixed Vegetables (bell peppers, cherry tomatoes, cucumbers), diced

1 tbsp Olive Oil

Salt and Pepper to taste

1 tbsp Fresh Cilantro, chopped

Instructions:

Mix quinoa and vegetables in a bowl.

Drizzle with olive oil and season with salt and pepper.

Garnish with fresh cilantro before serving.

Nutritional Information (per serving):

Calories: 220

Protein: 8g

Carbs: 30g

Fat: 8g

Notes

_____

_____

_____

_____

_____

_____

Apple Slices with Almond Butter

Preparation Time:	Cooking Time:	Servings:
5 minutes	**0 minutes**	**2**

Ingredients:

1 large Apple, washed and sliced   2 tbsp Almond Butter

Instructions:

Arrange apple slices on a plate.

Serve with almond butter for dipping.

Nutritional Information (per serving):

Calories: 200   Carbs: 25g

Protein: 5g   Fat: 11g

Notes

_____

_____

_____

_____

_____

_____

Vegetable Crudites with Tzatziki Sauce

Preparation Time:
10 minutes

Cooking Time:
0 minutes

Servings:
2

Ingredients:

1 cup Mixed Vegetables (carrots, celery, bell peppers), sliced

½ cup Homemade Tzatziki Sauce

Homemade Tzatziki Sauce:

- 1 cup Greek yogurt
- 1/2 cucumber, finely grated and drained
- 1 clove garlic, minced
- 1 tbsp fresh dill, chopped
- 1 tbsp Olive Oil
- Juice of 1/2 lemon
- Salt and Pepper to taste

Instructions:

Arrange vegetable slices on a plate.

For the tzatziki Sauce, combine all ingredients in a bowl and mix well. Chill in the refrigerator for at least 30 minutes before serving to allow flavors to meld.

Serve vegetable slices with tzatziki sauce for dipping.

Nutritional Information (per serving):

Calories: 100

Carbs: 10g

Protein: 3g

Fat: 5g

Notes

_____

_____

_____

_____

_____

_____

Spiced Pumpkin Seeds

Preparation Time:	Cooking Time:	Servings:
5 minutes	15 minutes	2

Ingredients:

½ cup Pumpkin Seeds, raw

1 tsp Olive Oil

¼ tsp Paprika

Salt to taste

Instructions:

Preheat oven to 350°F (180°C).

Toss pumpkin seeds with olive oil, paprika, and salt.

Spread on a baking sheet in a single layer.

Roast until golden brown, about 15 minutes, stirring occasionally.

Nutritional Information (per serving):

Calories: 180

Protein: 9g

Carbs: 3g

Fat: 16g

Notes

_____

_____

_____

_____

_____

_____

Cantaloupe and Prosciutto Bites

Preparation Time:	Cooking Time:	Servings:
10 minutes	0 minutes	2

Ingredients:

1 cup Cantaloupe, cut into bite-sized pieces

6 slices Prosciutto, halved

Instructions:

Wrap each piece of cantaloupe with a half slice of prosciutto.
Secure with a toothpick and serve as a refreshing and savory snack.

Nutritional Information (per serving):

Calories: 120

Carbs: 10g

Protein: 7g

Fat: 6g

Notes

_____

_____

_____

_____

_____

_____

8. Desserts to Indulge In

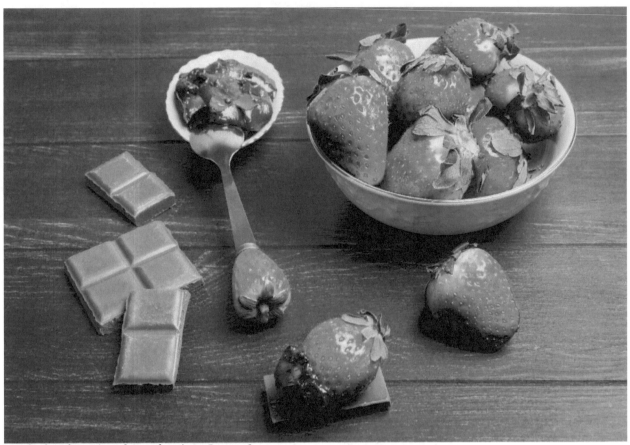

Dark Chocolate Dipped Strawberries – Page 108

Desserts in the realm of clean eating transform the ordinary finale of a meal into an extraordinary moment of healthy indulgence. Imagine concluding your day with desserts that feel like a treat, yet you're nurturing your body with every bite. It's not about deprivation; it's about celebrating natural sweetness and rich flavors.

Clean eating desserts are about savoring the natural sweetness of ingredients, enjoying the essence of each element, and feeling good about the treats you're consuming. They're about pleasure without compromise, sweetness without sacrifice.

Berry & Honey Yogurt Parfait

Preparation Time:	Cooking Time:	Servings:
10 minutes	0 minutes	2

Ingredients:

1 cup Mixed Berries (fresh or frozen)   2 tbsp Honey

1 cup Greek Yogurt   2 tbsp Granola

Instructions:

In glasses, layer Greek yogurt, mixed berries, honey, and granola.

Serve immediately or refrigerate until ready to serve.

Nutritional Information (per serving):

Calories: 220   Carbs: 32g

Protein: 12g   Fat: 5g

Notes

_____

_____

_____

_____

_____

_____

Baked Apple with Cinnamon and Walnuts

Preparation Time:	**Cooking Time:**	**Servings:**
10 minutes	30 minutes	2

Ingredients:

1 large Apple, cored   2 tbsp Walnuts, chopped

1 tsp Cinnamon   1 tbsp Honey

Instructions:

Preheat oven to 350°F (180°C).

Place apple in a baking dish and sprinkle with cinnamon and walnuts.

Drizzle honey over the top and bake for 30 minutes or until tender.

Nutritional Information (per serving):

Calories: 180   Carbs: 30g

Protein: 2g   Fat: 8g

Notes

_____

_____

_____

_____

_____

_____

Peach & Almond Smoothie

Preparation Time:	Cooking Time:	Servings:
5 minutes	**0 minutes**	**2**

Ingredients:

1 cup Peach slices (fresh or frozen)   1 tbsp Almond Butter

1 cup Almond Milk   1 tbsp Honey

Instructions:

Blend all ingredients until smooth.

Serve immediately.

Nutritional Information (per serving):

Calories: 160   Carbs: 20g

Protein: 3g   Fat: 9g

Notes

_____

_____

_____

_____

_____

_____

Dark Chocolate Dipped Strawberries

Preparation Time:
15 minutes

Cooking Time:
0 minutes

Servings:
2

Ingredients:

8 large Strawberries, washed and dried

2 oz Dark Chocolate (70% cocoa or higher)

Instructions:

Melt dark chocolate in a microwave-safe bowl in 30-second increments.

After dipping strawberries into melted chocolate, let them rest on parchment paper.

Nutritional Information (per serving):

Calories: 180

Carbs: 20g

Protein: 2g

Fat: 11g

Notes

_____

_____

_____

_____

_____

_____

Mango and Coconut Sorbet

Preparation Time:
10 minutes (plus
freezing time)

Cooking Time:
0 minutes

Servings:
2

Ingredients:

1 cup Mango, diced
½ cup Coconut Milk

1 tbsp Honey

Instructions:

Blend mango, coconut milk, and honey until smooth.

Freeze mixture in a shallow dish, stirring every 30 minutes, until set.

Nutritional Information (per serving):

Calories: 180
Protein: 1g

Carbs: 25g
Fat: 9g

Notes

_____

_____

_____

_____

_____

_____

Banana & Peanut Butter Bites

Preparation Time:
10 minutes

Cooking Time:
0 minutes

Servings:
2

Ingredients:

1 large Banana, sliced

2 tbsp Peanut Butter, unsweetened

Instructions:

Spread peanut butter on half of the banana slices and top with the other halves, creating sandwiches.

Freeze for at least 1 hour before serving.

Nutritional Information (per serving):

Calories: 190

Carbs: 25g

Protein: 5g

Fat: 9g

Notes

_____

_____

_____

_____

_____

_____

Blueberry & Lemon Chia Pudding

Preparation Time:	Cooking Time:	Servings:
10 minutes (plus soaking time)	0 minutes	2

Ingredients:

2 tbsp Chia Seeds

1 cup Almond Milk

½ cup Blueberries

1 tbsp Lemon Juice

1 tbsp Honey

Instructions:

Mix chia seeds with almond milk and let soak for at least 1 hour or overnight.
Mix in blueberries, lemon juice, and honey before serving.

Nutritional Information (per serving):

Calories: 160

Protein: 3g

Carbs: 23g

Fat: 7g

Notes

_____

_____

_____

_____

_____

_____

Pineapple & Mint Salad

Preparation Time:
10 minutes

Cooking Time:
0 minutes

Servings:
2

Ingredients:

1 cup Pineapple, diced

1 tbsp Fresh Mint, chopped

1 tbsp Honey

Instructions:

Mix pineapple and mint in a bowl.

Drizzle with honey and serve chilled.

Nutritional Information (per serving):

Calories: 100

Protein: 1g

Carbs: 25g

Fat: 0g

Notes

_____

_____

_____

_____

_____

_____

Sweet Potato & Cinnamon Cookies

Preparation Time:	Cooking Time:	Servings:
15 minutes	**15 minutes**	**2**

Ingredients:

1 cup Sweet Potato, cooked and mashed

1 cup Almond Flour

2 tbsp Coconut Oil, melted

1 tbsp Cinnamon

1 tbsp Honey

Instructions:

Preheat oven to 350°F (180°C).

Mix all ingredients to form a dough and shape into cookies on a baking sheet.

Bake for 15 minutes or until edges are golden.

Nutritional Information (per serving):

Calories: 250

Protein: 6g

Carbs: 25g

Fat: 15g

Notes

_____

_____

_____

_____

_____

_____

Raspberry & Almond Butter Smoothie Bowl

Preparation Time:	Cooking Time:	Servings:
10 minutes	0 minutes	2

Ingredients:

1 cup Raspberries (fresh or frozen)   1 tbsp Almond Butter

1 Banana   1 tbsp Granola

1 cup Almond Milk

Instructions:

Blend raspberries, banana, almond milk, and almond butter until smooth.

Pour into bowls and top with granola.

Nutritional Information (per serving):

Calories: 230

Protein: 5g   Fat: 10g

Carbs: 35g

Notes

_____

_____

_____

_____

_____

_____

Date & Nut Energy Balls

Preparation Time:	Cooking Time:	Servings:
15 minutes	0 minutes	2

Ingredients:

1 cup Dates, pitted

½ cup Mixed Nuts (almonds, walnuts, etc.)

1 tbsp Coconut Oil

1 tbsp Cocoa Powder

Instructions:

Process dates, nuts, coconut oil, and cocoa powder in a food processor until a dough forms. Roll into balls and refrigerate until set.

Nutritional Information (per serving):

Calories: 320

Protein: 6g

Carbs: 40g

Fat: 18g

Notes

_____
_____
_____
_____
_____
_____

Chocolate Avocado Mousse

Preparation Time:	Cooking Time:	Servings:
10 minutes	0 minutes	2

Ingredients:

1 Avocado, ripe

2 tbsp Cocoa Powder

1 tbsp Honey

½ tsp Vanilla Extract

Instructions:

Blend all ingredients until smooth.

Refrigerate for at least 1 hour before serving.

Nutritional Information (per serving):

Calories: 250

Protein: 3g

Carbs: 25g

Fat: 18g

Notes

_____

_____

_____

_____

_____

_____

Coconut & Pineapple Ice Pops

Preparation Time:
10 minutes (plus
freezing time)

Cooking Time:
0 minutes

Servings:
2

Ingredients:

1 cup Pineapple, diced   1 tbsp Honey
½ cup Coconut Milk

Instructions:

Blend pineapple, coconut milk, and honey until smooth.
Pour into ice pop molds and freeze until set.

Nutritional Information (per serving):

Calories: 160   Carbs: 20g
Protein: 1g   Fat: 9g

Notes

_____

_____

_____

_____

_____

_____

Mixed Berry & Oat Bars

Preparation Time:
15 minutes

Cooking Time:
20 minutes

Servings:
2

Ingredients:

1 cup Mixed Berries (fresh or frozen)

1 cup Rolled Oats

1 tbsp Honey

1 tbsp Coconut Oil

Instructions:

Preheat oven to 350°F (180°C).

Mix all ingredients and press into a small baking dish.

Bake for 20 minutes or until edges are golden.

Nutritional Information (per serving):

Calories: 260

Protein: 5g

Carbs: 35g

Fat: 12g

Notes

_____

_____

_____

_____

_____

_____

Kiwi & Mint Sorbet

Preparation Time:	Cooking Time:	Servings:
10 minutes (plus freezing time)	0 minutes	2

Ingredients:

2 Kiwis, peeled and diced

1 tbsp Fresh Mint, chopped

1 tbsp Honey

Instructions:

Blend kiwis, mint, and honey until smooth.

Freeze mixture in a shallow dish, stirring every 30 minutes, until set.

Nutritional Information (per serving):

Calories: 100

Protein: 1g

Carbs: 25g

Fat: 0g

Notes

_____

_____

_____

_____

_____

_____

9. Beverages to Refresh

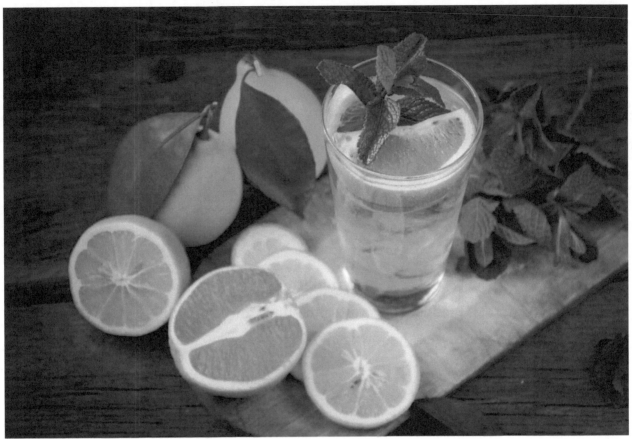

Citrus & Mint Infused Water – Page 124

Beverages in clean eating are like liquid gold, nourishing your body while pleasing your palate, without any artificial additives or excessive sugars. They're concoctions that hydrate, energize, and delight, made from the purest ingredients nature has to offer.

Clean eating beverages celebrate the natural flavors and innate goodness of ingredients, providing hydration and enjoyment without any guilt. They're about quenching your thirst and nurturing your body, one sip at a time.

Strawberry Basil Lemonade

Preparation Time:	Cooking Time:	Servings:
10 minutes	0 minutes	2

Ingredients:

1 cup Strawberries, halved

1 Lemon, juiced

2 tbsp Fresh Basil, chopped

2 tbsp Honey

4 cups Water

Instructions:

Blend strawberries, lemon juice, basil, and honey until smooth.

Strain and mix with water.

Serve over ice.

Nutritional Information (per serving):

Calories: 80

Protein: 0g

Carbs: 21g

Fat: 0g

Notes

_____

_____

_____

_____

_____

_____

Cucumber Mint Cooler

Preparation Time:
10 minutes

Cooking Time:
0 minutes

Servings:
2

Ingredients:

½ Cucumber, sliced

4 sprigs of Fresh Mint

1 Lime, juiced

1 tbsp Honey

4 cups Sparkling Water

Instructions:

Muddle cucumber, mint, lime juice, and honey in a pitcher.

Add sparkling water and serve over ice.

Nutritional Information (per serving):

Calories: 40

Protein: 0g

Carbs: 10g

Fat: 0g

Notes

_____

_____

_____

_____

_____

_____

Vanilla Almond Milkshake

Preparation Time:	Cooking Time:	Servings:
5 minutes	0 minutes	2

Ingredients:

2 cups Almond Milk   1 tbsp Honey

1 tsp Vanilla Extract   1 cup Ice

Instructions:

Blend all ingredients until smooth.

Serve immediately.

Nutritional Information (per serving):

Calories: 90   Carbs: 15g

Protein: 1g   Fat: 3g

Notes

_____

_____

_____

_____

_____

_____

Citrus & Mint Infused Water

Preparation Time: **Cooking Time:**   **Servings:**

5 minutes   0 minutes   2

Ingredients:

1 Orange, sliced

1 Lemon, sliced

1 Lime, sliced

4 sprigs of Fresh Mint

4 cups Water

Instructions:

Combine all the ingredients in a pitcher.

Refrigerate for at least 1 hour before serving.

Nutritional Information (per serving):

Calories: 30

Protein: 0g

Carbs: 10g

Fat: 0g

Notes

_____

_____

_____

_____

_____

_____

Pineapple Ginger Smoothie

Preparation Time:

5 minutes

Cooking Time:

0 minutes

Servings:

2

Ingredients:

1 cup Pineapple chunks

1 tsp Fresh Ginger, grated

1 cup Coconut Water

1 tbsp Honey

Instructions:

Blend all ingredients until smooth.

Serve immediately.

Nutritional Information (per serving):

Calories: 90

Protein: 1g

Carbs: 22g

Fat: 0g

Notes

_____

_____

_____

_____

_____

_____

Berry Green Tea Smoothie

Preparation Time:
5 minutes

Cooking Time:
0 minutes

Servings:
2

Ingredients:

1 cup Mixed Berries (like strawberries, blueberries, raspberries)

1 cup Brewed Green Tea, cooled

1 tbsp Honey

1 cup Ice

Instructions:

Blend all ingredients until smooth.

Serve immediately.

Nutritional Information (per serving):

Calories: 70

Protein: 0g

Carbs: 17g

Fat: 0g

Notes

_____

_____

_____

_____

_____

_____

Cherry Lime Sparkler

Preparation Time:	**Cooking Time:**	**Servings:**
10 minutes	0 minutes	2

Ingredients:

1 cup Cherries, pitted

1 Lime, juiced

1 tbsp Honey

4 cups Sparkling Water

Instructions:

Blend cherries, lime juice, and honey until smooth.

Strain and mix with sparkling water.

Serve over ice.

Nutritional Information (per serving):

Calories: 70

Protein: 1g

Carbs: 18g

Fat: 0g

Notes

_____

_____

_____

_____

_____

_____

Spiced Almond Latte

Preparation Time:
5 minutes

Cooking Time:
5 minutes

Servings:
2

Ingredients:

2 cups Almond Milk

1 tsp Cinnamon

½ tsp Nutmeg

1 tbsp Honey

2 shots of Espresso (or 1 cup Brewed Coffee)

Instructions:

Heat almond milk with cinnamon, nutmeg, and honey until hot but not boiling.

Pour over espresso or coffee.

Serve immediately.

Nutritional Information (per serving):

Calories: 80

Protein: 1g

Carbs: 14g

Fat: 3g

Notes

_____

_____

_____

_____

_____

_____

Mango Coconut Water Smoothie

Preparation Time:
5 minutes

Cooking Time:
0 minutes

Servings:
2

Ingredients:

1 Mango, peeled and diced

1 cup Coconut Water

1 tbsp Honey

1 cup Ice

Instructions:

Blend all ingredients until smooth.

Serve immediately.

Nutritional Information (per serving):

Calories: 100

Protein: 1g

Carbs: 25g

Fat: 0g

Notes

_____

_____

_____

_____

_____

_____

Apple Cinnamon Infused Water

Preparation Time:

5 minutes

Cooking Time:

0 minutes

Servings:

2

Ingredients:

1 Apple, sliced

1 Cinnamon Stick

4 cups Water

Instructions:

Combine all the ingredients in a pitcher.

Refrigerate for at least 1 hour before serving.

Nutritional Information (per serving):

Calories: 50

Protein: 0g

Carbs: 14g

Fat: 0g

Notes

_____

_____

_____

_____

_____

_____

10. Clean Eating Lifestyle Tips

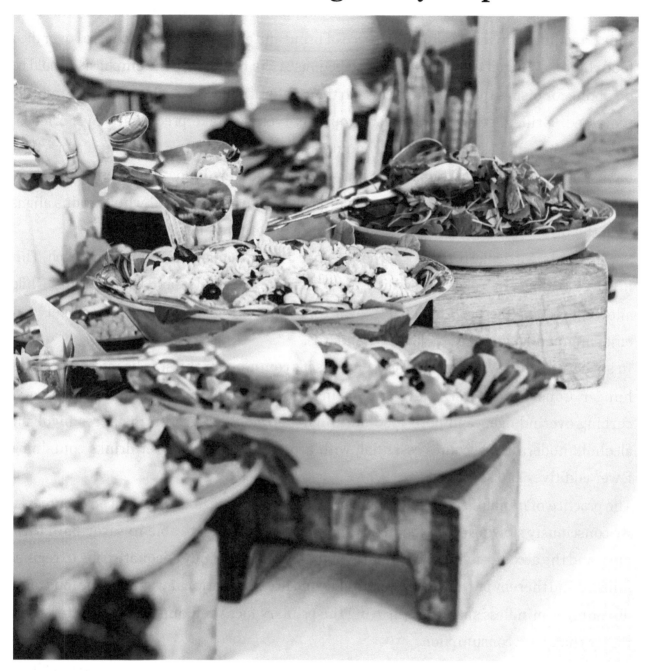

Eating Out and Social Events

Navigating social events and dining out while maintaining a commitment to a clean eating lifestyle can often present challenges, yet with strategic approaches and careful planning, these social occasions can be thoroughly enjoyed without compromising core dietary principles. Preparation is undeniably key; conducting research in advance of attending a restaurant or social event can yield valuable insights into menu options, thereby enabling individuals to pre-plan their meals in alignment with their dietary preferences. This proactive strategy extends to contacting the restaurant or event host beforehand to inquire about specific menu items, their preparation methods, and the potential for special, diet-compliant requests, an approach that most establishments are inclined to accommodate, thus providing individuals with both peace of mind and a greater sense of control over their food choices. When it comes to making selections at the restaurant, the emphasis should be on opting for dishes that remain as close to their natural state as possible and are minimally processed. Grilled, steamed, or roasted options typically take precedence over fried or creamy dishes, and asking for sauces and dressings to be served on the side is a practical tactic for ensuring moderation in consumption and avoiding hidden calories or additives. Furthermore, prioritizing the intake of lean proteins, vegetables, and whole grains aligns with the nutritional balance that is central to clean eating principles.

Social events, particularly those with buffet-style dining, demand a strategic approach. This involves loading one's plate predominantly with fruits, vegetables, and lean proteins, while allowing for smaller portions of less healthy options, thus striking a balance between enjoyment and adherence to dietary standards.

In such settings, staying hydrated is crucial, as it's common for thirst to be misconstrued as hunger. Consuming water before and during the event aids in maintaining satiety and curbing overindulgence in both food and high-calorie beverages. In instances involving alcohol, moderation becomes essential, with a preference for simpler drinks containing fewer additives and sugars.

The practice of mindful eating takes on increased significance in these social environments. By consciously slowing down food consumption, individuals are able to savor both their meal and the accompanying social interactions, allowing the body adequate time to register fullness and thereby prevent overeating. Engaging in conversations away from the food table discourages mindless snacking, ensuring the primary focus remains on social interaction rather than food consumption.

Despite these challenges, it's imperative to adopt a flexible attitude. Clean eating is not about attaining perfection, and occasional indulgences are a natural aspect of a balanced lifestyle. The objective remains to make the most informed and healthful choices possible while relishing the social interactions, without permitting food-related anxieties to detract from the event's enjoyment.

In conclusion, the ultimate goal is to partake in and savor social occasions and dining experiences without deviating significantly from clean eating principles. Through adequate preparation, mindfulness, and informed decision-making, individuals can easily fully engage in and deriving pleasure from eating out and social events.

Staying Motivated in Clean Eating Journey

Staying motivated in your clean eating journey necessitates a multifaceted approach, intertwining the establishment of realistic goals, acknowledgment of progress, leveraging social support, and cultivating resilience to overcome inevitable challenges. Initiating this journey requires the articulation of clear, specific objectives that are realistically attainable, such as integrating a designated quantity of fruits and vegetables into your daily regimen, curtailing the intake of processed foods, or committing to cooking homemade meals multiple times a week. It's pivotal to avoid the pitfall of setting overly ambitious goals, as they can precipitate frustration and diminish motivation. Concurrently, it's vital to celebrate the small victories along the way.

Sharing your aspirations for clean eating with friends, family, or engaging with a community of like-minded individuals can provide a reservoir of encouragement, shared wisdom, and even foster healthy competition. This network becomes a cornerstone of motivation, especially during moments of waning willpower. Furthermore, comprehending the profound influence of dietary choices on personal health, holistic well-being, and even environmental stewardship can act as a potent motivator.

Visual cues are also a powerful tool; maintaining tangible reminders of your dietary objectives and the underlying reasons for pursuing this lifestyle can serve as constant sources of inspiration.

The path will undoubtedly present challenges, including social engagements, travel, or simply hectic schedules. Anticipating these obstacles and devising strategies to navigate them is crucial. Attuning to your body's responses to clean eating—such as heightened energy, mood enhancement, improved sleep patterns, or potential weight loss—also provides tangible incentives to persevere.

Additionally, establishing a reward system that eschews food-based incentives can be effective; rewarding milestones with a new book, a therapeutic massage, or a day dedicated to a cherished hobby can reinforce positive behavior. Periodic reflection on your journey offers profound insights into the strategies that are effective and those necessitating reevaluation, thereby facilitating continued motivation and adjustment of your approach as needed.

It's imperative to recognize that clean eating is akin to a marathon, not a sprint; it's a gradual process of instilling enduring modifications to your dietary habits, culminating in a healthier, more fulfilled version of yourself.

11. Conclusion

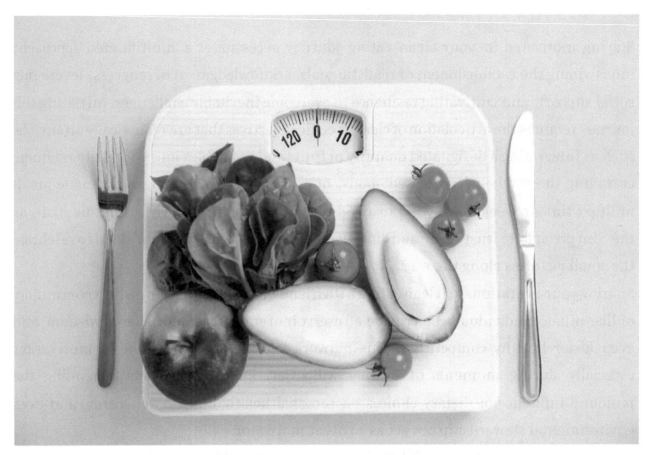

Recapitulation of Clean Eating Benefits

Recapitulating the myriad benefits of clean eating, it's imperative to emphasize that this regimen is not merely a diet but a transformative approach that profoundly impacts diverse aspects of human health and holistic well-being. Embarking on a clean eating journey primarily fortifies overall health, as the body revels in a bounty of essential nutrients obtained from unadulterated, minimally processed foods, thereby bolstering immune competency and optimizing organ functionality. The intrinsic richness of whole foods in vital vitamins, minerals, and antioxidants plays a cardinal role in shielding the body from chronic ailments, including cardiovascular diseases, diabetes, and various forms of cancer.

A notable surge in energy levels is a welcome corollary of clean eating, attributable to the equilibrium in blood sugar levels engendered by the consumption of whole, unprocessed foods. This starkly contrasts with the erratic energy fluctuations commonly triggered by refined sugars and carbohydrates. This newfound metabolic stability not only fuels physical vigor but also augments cognitive acumen, manifesting in enhanced concentration and a pervasive sense of alertness. Furthermore, the realm of weight management becomes less daunting, as clean eating inherently precludes processed foods laden with empty calories, thereby naturally mitigating caloric excess and simplifying the dual objectives of weight reduction and sustenance of a healthy weight.

Digestive health reaps substantial benefits from the fiber-laden constituents of clean eating, such as whole grains, fruits, and vegetables. Sufficient fiber consumption is pivotal for consistent bowel regularity and the cultivation of a harmonious gut microbiome, both of which are quintessential for digestive prosperity and systemic health. Moreover, the potent anti-inflammatory virtues of numerous whole foods, particularly those abundant in omega-3 fatty acids and antioxidants, are instrumental in diminishing inflammation, a ubiquitous precursor to a plethora of health quandaries, ranging from arthritic afflictions to cardiovascular anomalies.

The psychological dividends of clean eating, though less conspicuous, are equally consequential. The calibre of dietary intake exerts a profound influence on neurological vitality, with repercussions for emotional disposition and susceptibility to depressive states. Diets replete with nutrients correlate with an uplifted mood, attenuated anxiety indicators, and an overarching sense of psychological well-being. An ancillary boon of clean eating is the enhancement of sleep quality, especially when the dietary repertoire includes foods endowed with nutrients that foster sleep, such as magnesium and calcium.

The propensity for a longer life attributable to clean eating is incontrovertible, given its comprehensive health advantages, diminution of disease susceptibility, and promotion of weight equilibrium, collectively contributing to an extended lifespan. The environmental ramifications of clean eating are also salient, given the predilection for locally procured, organically cultivated produce, which mitigates the carbon footprint associated with conventional food production and logistics, thereby bolstering local agricultural sectors and endorsing ecological sustainability.

From an economic perspective, clean eating can precipitate a reduction in healthcare expenditures over the long term. Despite the potentially higher initial investment in organic or whole foods, the ensuing health dividends can translate into diminished medical expenses, infrequent healthcare consultations, and a lesser reliance on medicinal interventions, culminating in substantial financial savings.

In essence, clean eating is a panacea of sorts, bestowing a plethora of benefits that transcend the physical and permeate every facet of human existence, from corporeal vitality to environmental conservation, emphatically affirming its indispensability as a cornerstone of a superior, health-oriented lifestyle.

Encouragement and Final Thoughts on Clean Eating

Embarking on a clean eating journey signifies more than a mere dietary change; it's a laudable commitment to enhancing personal health and contributing to a broader ethos of environmental sustainability and conscientious food consumption practices. This path transcends restrictive, ephemeral dieting trends, representing instead a perpetual commitment to judicious, health-promoting choices, fundamentally centered around the nourishment of one's body with unrefined, natural foods and an inherent respect for the environment that yields these resources.

A critical ethos to internalize is that the pursuit of perfection is secondary to the pursuit of consistency. Inevitable are the moments when deviations from the established plan occur, but these should not be deterrents. Instead, the focus should be on the resilience to realign with the foundational principles of clean eating and the wisdom to extract learning from every experience. The journey is undulating, replete with both triumphs and less successful moments, yet every step and decision coalesce to contribute indispensably to holistic well-being. It's pivotal to recognize that this journey is not a solitary one. A burgeoning global community of advocates for clean eating exists, teeming with diverse experiences and insights. Engaging with this community, exchanging narratives, and drawing learning from one another can furnish not only sustained motivation but also a rich tapestry of perspectives and pragmatic guidance. Furthermore, the realm of nutrition is ever-evolving, with fresh research perennially emerging. Remaining abreast of these scientific advancements is crucial.

Progress on this journey merits recognition and celebration, irrespective of scale. Every healthful choice epitomizes a triumph, deserving acknowledgment. This personal journey, moreover, possesses the potential to catalyze wider change, inspiring acquaintances and loved ones to echo these healthful choices, thereby creating a positive ripple effect. Anticipate tangible enhancements in physical health manifesting as heightened vitality, improved digestive function, and potential weight regulation, among other benefits. Equally profound are the mental and emotional dividends, including mood stabilization, enhanced cognitive clarity, and an elevated sense of overall well-being.

Permit food to transcend its role as mere physical sustenance, allowing it to nourish the soul profoundly. Undertake this journey with unwavering positivity and receptiveness, permitting the tenets of clean eating to steer you towards an existence marked by enhanced health and happiness.

12. Bonus: Meal Plan

Meal planning stands paramount in clean eating, acting as a nutritional compass, steering individuals toward health goals while infusing simplicity and pleasure into the eating experience, transforming it from a mere task to a gratifying journey toward a vibrant life. This proactive approach addresses typical clean eating obstacles like time restrictions and monotony, easing the shift to nutritious habits and fostering a lasting allegiance to a wholesome lifestyle, thereby unlocking the extensive rewards of balanced nutrition. Recognizing meal planning's role in clean eating is essential; it enhances efficiency and time stewardship by streamlining grocery shopping and meal preparation, curtails food wastage, and alleviates the daily quandary of meal selection. It guarantees nutritional equilibrium in every meal, aligning with wellness aspirations, and is economical, circumventing impulsive purchases and adhering to budgetary constraints. Prepared meals diminish the temptation for processed alternatives, fortifying the resolve for healthful choices.

Effective meal planning involves evaluating dietary needs and predilections, devising a diverse weekly menu, and formulating an organized grocery list. It necessitates dedicated preparation time to preclude eleventh-hour pressures and precise portioning to obviate excess consumption and wastage. Clean eating meal plans should concentrate on unprocessed items, incorporating an array of foodstuffs and cooking styles, and adjusting portions per energy requirements, with an element of flexibility for unforeseen adjustments. Novices should initiate small, perhaps focusing on singular meal times, progressively expanding to more intricate preparations. Utilize batch cooking for convenience, invest in quality storage for food longevity, and plan assorted menus to avert dietary ennui. Employ kitchen gadgets to expedite and simplify tasks, pre-portion to regulate nutritional intake, label containers for organization and freshness, and include meals conducive to freezing, ensuring constant availability of wholesome options.

MY 30-Day MEAL PLAN

Day 1:
Breakfast: Sunrise Smoothie Bowl
Lunch: Herb-Crusted Chicken Salad
Dinner: Herb-Crusted Chicken with Sweet Potato Mash
Snack: Carrot and Cucumber Sticks with Hummus
Dessert: Berry & Honey Yogurt Parfait
Beverage: Strawberry Basil Lemonade
Total Nutritional Information:
Calories: 1460
Protein: 88g
Carbs: 139g
Fat: 59g

Day 2:
Breakfast: Energizing Oat Pancakes
Lunch: Refreshing Cucumber Avocado Salad
Dinner: Lemon-Herb Tilapia with Asparagus
Snack: Roasted Sweet Potato Wedges
Dessert: Baked Apple with Cinnamon and Walnuts
Beverage: Cucumber Mint Cooler
Total Nutritional Information:
Calories: 1310
Protein: 54g
Carbs: 161g
Fat: 56g

Day 3:
Breakfast: Savory Veggie Omelette
Lunch: Spaghetti Squash with Tomato Basil Sauce
Dinner: Herb-Crusted Tilapia with Quinoa
Snack: Zucchini and Corn Sauté
Dessert: Peach & Almond Smoothie
Beverage: Vanilla Almond Milkshake
Total Nutritional Information:
Calories: 1240
Protein: 57g
Carbs: 128g
Fat: 56g

Day 4:
Breakfast: Almond Butter and Banana Sandwich
Lunch: Zesty Lemon Tilapia
Dinner: Mushroom and Spinach Stuffed Chicken Breast
Snack: Crispy Kale Chips
Dessert: Dark Chocolate Dipped Strawberries
Beverage: Citrus & Mint Infused Water
Total Nutritional Information:
Calories: 1270
Protein: 80g
Carbs: 103g
Fat: 66g

Day 5:
Breakfast: Green Power Smoothie
Lunch: Mushroom & Spinach Frittata
Dinner: Spicy Radish Tacos
Snack: Cherry Tomato and Mozzarella Salad
Dessert: Mango and Coconut Sorbet
Beverage: Pineapple Ginger Smoothie
Total Nutritional Information:
Calories: 1290
Protein: 35g
Carbs: 164g
Fat: 56g

Day 6:
Breakfast: Avocado Toast with Poached Eggs
Lunch: Hearty Lentil Soup
Dinner: Cauliflower Steak with Chimichurri Sauce
Snack: Mixed Nuts and Seeds
Dessert: Banana & Peanut Butter Bites
Beverage: Berry Green Tea Smoothie
Total Nutritional Information:
Calories: 1550
Protein: 66g
Carbs: 171g
Fat: 81g

Day 7:
Breakfast: Mango Coconut Smoothie
Lunch: Spicy Pineapple Chicken
Dinner: Grilled Salmon with Avocado Salsa
Snack: Baked Radish Chips
Dessert: Blueberry & Lemon Chia Pudding
Beverage: Cherry Lime Sparkler
Total Nutritional Information:
Calories: 1510
Protein: 100g
Carbs: 136g
Fat: 77g

Day 8:
Breakfast: Berry Quinoa Breakfast Bowl
Lunch: Grilled Veggie Platter
Dinner: Sweet and Spicy Baked Pineapple Chicken
Snack: Oven-Roasted Brussel Sprouts
Dessert: Pineapple & Mint Salad
Beverage: Spiced Almond Latte
Total Nutritional Information:
Calories: 1390
Protein: 73g
Carbs: 194g
Fat: 49g

Day 9:
Breakfast: Fruity Chia Pudding
Lunch: Baked Sweet Potato with Avocado Salsa
Dinner: Roasted Beet and Goat Cheese Salad
Snack: Quinoa and Vegetable Salad
Dessert: Sweet Potato & Cinnamon Cookies
Beverage: Mango Coconut Water Smoothie
Total Nutritional Information:
Calories: 1500
Protein: 27g
Carbs: 188g
Fat: 63g

Day 10:
Breakfast: Zesty Veggie Scramble
Lunch: Spinach and Feta Stuffed Chicken
Dinner: Cajun Spiced Sweet Potato Fries
Snack: Apple Slices with Almond Butter
Dessert: Raspberry & Almond Butter Smoothie Bowl
Beverage: Apple Cinnamon Infused Water
Total Nutritional Information:
Calories: 1540
Protein: 73g
Carbs: 145g
Fat: 82g

Day 11:
Breakfast: Berry Nutty Oatmeal
Lunch: Lemon Herb Quinoa Salad
Dinner: Mango Avocado Salsa Chicken
Snack: Vegetable Crudites with Tzatziki Sauce
Dessert: Date & Nut Energy Balls
Beverage: Strawberry Basil Lemonade
Total Nutritional Information:
Calories: 1520
Protein: 66g
Carbs: 186g
Fat: 71g

Day 12:
Breakfast: Protein-Packed Avocado Toast
Lunch: Honey Mustard Grilled Salmon
Dinner: Zesty Lemon Asparagus Shrimp
Snack: Spiced Pumpkin Seeds
Dessert: Chocolate Avocado Mousse
Beverage: Cucumber Mint Cooler
Total Nutritional Information:
Calories: 1390
Protein: 85g
Carbs: 104g
Fat: 83g

Day 13:
Breakfast: Hearty Veggie Frittata
Lunch: Vegetable Stir-Fry with Brown Rice
Dinner: Butternut Squash and Spinach Risotto
Snack: Cantaloupe and Prosciutto Bites
Dessert: Coconut & Pineapple Ice Pops
Beverage: Vanilla Almond Milkshake
Total Nutritional Information:
Calories: 1380
Protein: 40g
Carbs: 204g
Fat: 51g

Day 14:
Breakfast: Refreshing Cucumber Melon Smoothie
Lunch: Spaghetti Squash Primavera
Dinner: Mediterranean Chickpea Salad
Snack: Carrot and Cucumber Sticks with Hummus
Dessert: Mixed Berry & Oat Bars
Beverage: Citrus & Mint Infused Water
Total Nutritional Information:
Calories: 1190
Protein: 29g
Carbs: 175g
Fat: 41g

Day 15:
Breakfast: Energizing Fruit and Nut Yogurt Parfait
Lunch: Creamy Avocado and Spinach Pasta
Dinner: Balsamic Glazed Salmon
Snack: Roasted Sweet Potato Wedges
Dessert: Kiwi & Mint Sorbet
Beverage: Pineapple Ginger Smoothie
Total Nutritional Information:
Calories: 1520
Protein: 50g
Carbs: 202g
Fat: 62g

Day 16:
Breakfast: Savory Spinach and Mushroom Oatmeal
Lunch: Apple Walnut Salad with Grilled Chicken
Dinner: Stuffed Bell Peppers
Snack: Zucchini and Corn Sauté
Dessert: Berry & Honey Yogurt Parfait
Beverage: Berry Green Tea Smoothie
Total Nutritional Information:
Calories: 1510
Protein: 67g
Carbs: 187g
Fat: 58g

Day 17:
Breakfast: Protein-Packed Quinoa Breakfast Bowl
Lunch: Spicy Avocado Tuna Salad
Dinner: Roasted Vegetable Medley
Snack: Crispy Kale Chips
Dessert: Baked Apple with Cinnamon and Walnuts
Beverage: Cherry Lime Sparkler
Total Nutritional Information:
Calories: 1290
Protein: 66g
Carbs: 138g
Fat: 54g

Day 18:
Breakfast: Sunrise Smoothie Bowl
Lunch: Roasted Vegetable and Lentil Salad
Dinner: Grilled Lemon Herb Chicken
Snack: Cherry Tomato and Mozzarella Salad
Dessert: Peach & Almond Smoothie
Beverage: Spiced Almond Latte
Total Nutritional Information:
Calories: 1370
Protein: 70g
Carbs: 143g
Fat: 57g

Day 19:
Breakfast: Energizing Oat Pancakes
Lunch: Herb-Infused Baked Salmon
Dinner: Sweet Potato and Black Bean Bowl
Snack: Mixed Nuts and Seeds
Dessert: Dark Chocolate Dipped Strawberries
Beverage: Mango Coconut Water Smoothie
Total Nutritional Information:
Calories: 1640
Protein: 77g
Carbs: 167g
Fat: 92g

Day 20:
Breakfast: Savory Veggie Omelette
Lunch: Ginger-Soy Infused Steamed Cod
Dinner: Butternut Squash and Kale Risotto
Snack: Baked Radish Chips
Dessert: Mango and Coconut Sorbet
Beverage: Apple Cinnamon Infused Water
Total Nutritional Information:
Calories: 1290
Protein: 61g
Carbs: 155g
Fat: 47g

Day 21:
Breakfast: Green Power Smoothie
Lunch: Spicy Pineapple Chicken
Dinner: Grilled Salmon with Avocado Salsa
Snack: Apple Slices with Almond Butter
Dessert: Raspberry & Almond Butter Smoothie Bowl
Beverage: Strawberry Basil Lemonade
Total Nutritional Information:
Calories: 1440
Protein: 69g
Carbs: 182g
Fat: 60g

Day 22:
Breakfast: Almond Butter and Banana Sandwich
Lunch: Spaghetti Squash with Tomato Basil Sauce
Dinner: Cajun Spiced Sweet Potato Fries
Snack: Quinoa and Vegetable Salad
Dessert: Sweet Potato & Cinnamon Cookies
Beverage: Cucumber Mint Cooler
Total Nutritional Information:
Calories: 1390
Protein: 26g
Carbs: 245g
Fat: 47g

Day 23:
Breakfast: Mango Coconut Smoothie
Lunch: Grilled Veggie Platter
Dinner: Lemon-Herb Tilapia with Asparagus
Snack: Oven-Roasted Brussel Sprouts
Dessert: Blueberry & Lemon Chia Pudding
Beverage: Vanilla Almond Milkshake
Total Nutritional Information:
Calories: 1190
Protein: 36g
Carbs: 147g
Fat: 51g

Day 24:
Breakfast: Berry Quinoa Breakfast Bowl
Lunch: Spinach and Feta Stuffed Chicken
Dinner: Roasted Beet and Goat Cheese Salad
Snack: Vegetable Crudites with Tzatziki Sauce
Dessert: Pineapple & Mint Salad
Beverage: Citrus & Mint Infused Water
Total Nutritional Information:
Calories: 1320
Protein: 77g
Carbs: 113g
Fat: 57g

Day 25:
Breakfast: Fruity Chia Pudding
Lunch: Lemon Herb Quinoa Salad
Dinner: Sweet and Spicy Baked Pineapple Chicken
Snack: Carrot and Cucumber Sticks with Hummus
Dessert: Coconut & Pineapple Ice Pops
Beverage: Pineapple Ginger Smoothie
Total Nutritional Information:
Calories: 1290
Protein: 38g
Carbs: 185g
Fat: 41g

Day 26:
Breakfast: Zesty Veggie Scramble
Lunch: Honey Mustard Grilled Salmon
Dinner: Butternut Squash and Spinach Risotto
Snack: Crispy Kale Chips
Dessert: Berry & Honey Yogurt Parfait
Beverage: Berry Green Tea Smoothie
Total Nutritional Information:
Calories: 1520
Protein: 82g
Carbs: 185g
Fat: 54g

Day 27:
Breakfast: Berry Nutty Oatmeal
Lunch: Spicy Avocado Tuna Salad
Dinner: Grilled Lemon Herb Chicken
Snack: Zucchini and Corn Sauté
Dessert: Date & Nut Energy Balls
Beverage: Cherry Lime Sparkler
Total Nutritional Information:
Calories: 1520
Protein: 77g
Carbs: 163g
Fat: 71g

Day 28:
Breakfast: Protein-Packed Avocado Toast
Lunch: Vegetable Stir-Fry with Brown Rice
Dinner: Mediterranean Chickpea Salad
Snack: Spiced Pumpkin Seeds
Dessert: Chocolate Avocado Mousse
Beverage: Spiced Almond Latte
Total Nutritional Information:
Calories: 1470
Protein: 49g
Carbs: 178g
Fat: 72g

Day 29:
Breakfast: Hearty Veggie Frittata
Lunch: Apple Walnut Salad with Grilled Chicken
Dinner: Roasted Vegetable Medley
Snack: Cherry Tomato and Mozzarella Salad
Dessert: Peach & Almond Smoothie
Beverage: Mango Coconut Water Smoothie
Total Nutritional Information:
Calories: 1370
Protein: 72g
Carbs: 133g
Fat: 63g

Day 30:
Breakfast: Refreshing Cucumber Melon Smoothie
Lunch: Herb-Infused Baked Salmon
Dinner: Sweet Potato and Black Bean Bowl
Snack: Mixed Nuts and Seeds
Dessert: Dark Chocolate Dipped Strawberries
Beverage: Apple Cinnamon Infused Water

Total Nutritional Information:
Calories: 1510
Protein: 69g
Carbs: 143g
Fat: 82g

13. A to Z Recipes

Made in United States
Troutdale, OR
10/04/2024

23309492R00084